S
ALLE ZEIT WACH
1842

G. Staehler · S. Pomer (Eds.)

Contemporary Research on Renal Cell Carcinoma

Basic and Clinical Developments

With 27 Tables and 61 Figures, 3 in Color

Springer-Verlag
Berlin Heidelberg New York London Paris
Tokyo Hong Kong Barcelona Budapest

Professor Dr. med. GERD STAEHLER
PD Dr. med. SIGMUND POMER

Chirurgische Universitätsklinik
Abteilung Urologie und Poliklinik
Im Neuenheimer Feld 110
D-69120 Heidelberg, Germany

ISBN-13: 978-3-642-78611-2 e-ISBN-13: 978-3-642-78609-9
DOI: 10.1007/978-3-642-78609-9

Library of Congress Cataloging-in-Publication Data. Contemporary research on renal cell carcinoma: basic and clinical developments/G. Staehler, S. Pomer, eds. p. cm. Includes bibliographical references and index. ISBN 3-540-57375-5 – ISBN 0-387-57375-5 1. Renal cell carcinoma. 2. Metastasis. I. Staehler, G. (Gerd) II. Pomer, S. (Sigmund) [DNLM: 1. Carcinoma, Renal Cell – physiopathology. 2. Carcinoma, Renal Cell – therapy. 3. Kidney Neoplasms – physiopathology. 4. Kidney Neoplasms – therapy. WJ 358 C761 1993] RC280.K5C66 1993 616.99'461 – dc20 DNLM/DLC for Library of Congress 93–23588

Softcover reprint of the hardcover 1st edition 1994

Typesetting: Macmillan India Ltd., Bangalore 25
21/3130/SPS – 5 4 3 2 1 0 – Printed on acid-free paper

Preface

The management of advanced renal cell carcinoma is still problematic. Surgery, although the therapy of choice for locally advanced renal tumors, is still controversial as the treatment for metastases. The role of surgery in the management of patients with pulmonary, bony, and liver metastasis is one of the subject matters discussed in this book. Our results with series of patients undergoing resection of metastases from the lung, bone, and liver show that surgery may be appropriate in selected patients with a good performance status, although most of them certainly cannot be cured by this procedure alone, i.e., in the absence of effective adjuvant therapies.

As recent developments show, new strategies for immunotherapy of renal cell carcinoma represent a modest advance over traditional approaches in the treatment of this cancer, such as chemo- and radiotherapy. Clinical trials employing recombinant interferon-α and interleukin 2 produced response rates in up to 30% of patients treated, as evidenced by the European Immunotherapy Trials Program. The adverse reactions and the lack of efficacy in the majority of patients warrants the search for new immunotherapeutic approaches.

Our understanding of the molecular and cellular events connected with the malignant transformation of renal cell carcinoma is growing. Molecular studies have identified a basis for familial renal cancer, which in some cases occurs with features of von Hippel-Lindau disease. Abnormalities involving chromosome 3 have been described in nonpapillary carcinomas, implying that a tumor suppressor gene absence or inactivation may be the key initial event in the carcinogenesis of the heritable and sporadic forms of this neoplasm. Genetic changes on chromosomes 5 and 14 associated with progression of nonpapillary renal cancers have been described. The molecular characterization of papillary renal cell carcinoma as a distinct pathological entity has led to a new classification of renal tumors.

Hopefully, these developments will create a basis for more effective treatment of renal cell carcinoma in the future.

Heidelberg,
January 1994

G. Staehler
S. Pomer

Contents

I Clinical Research

Contributors

Addresses are given at the beginning of the respective contribution

I Clinical Research

The Role of Nephrectomy in Metastatic Renal Cell Carcinoma

E.A. Klein

Introduction

Radical nephrectomy is well established as the standard treatment for localized renal cell carcinoma. Nephrectomy is the only known curative therapy for this tumor. The role of radical nephrectomy in the management of metastatic renal cell carcinoma is controversial and has come under increased scrutiny in the past several years with the development of immunotherapy, which has the potential to cure systemic renal cell carcinoma. Thus, immunotherapy combined with radical nephrectomy has the potential to cure patients with metastatic disease.

The rationale for radical nephrectomy in the face of metastatic disease can be divided into therapeutic and adjunctive indications. Therapeutic indications include nephrectomy to help induce spontaneous regression of low-volume metastases, concomitantly at the time of excision of solitary metastases, in order to harvest tumor-infiltrating lymphocytes (TILs) or to consolidate clinical response following treatment with systemic chemotherapy or immunotherapy. The adjunctive indications for nephrectomy in this setting include palliation of local symptoms and improvement of the response to systemic immunotherapy prior to treatment. Other theoretical indications include preventing the development of new metastases and the prevention of future local symptoms and paraneoplastic syndromes.

There is some evidence in the literature suggesting that nephrectomy in the presence of metastatic cancer may improve overall survival [1–4] (Table 1). Although these data suggest a beneficial effect for patients undergoing nephrectomy, it is likely that only those patients with good performance status and minimal local disease were operated on in these series, and that patient selection factors could account for the apparent beneficial outcome. More recent evidence suggests that in patients matched for overall tumor burden those undergoing nephrectomy also had improved survival [5] (Table 2). This study also suggested an improved survival in patients with primary tumors less than 10 cm in size at the time of treatment. While these series are suggestive of an improvement in

Section of Urologic Oncology, Cleveland Clinic Foundation, 9500 Euclid Avenue, Cleveland, OH 44195, USA

Table 1. Nephrectomy (NX) in metastatic RCC: effect on survival (modified from [15])

Reference	NX	*n*	1 year %	3 years %	5 years %
Johnson et al. [1]	–	50	22	0	0
	+	43	36	11	0
Klugo et al. [2]	–	64	12	9	3
	+	37	49	24	11
Montie et al. [3]	–	16	0	0	0
	+	48	25	9	2
Patel and Lavengood [4]	–	25	9	4	4
	+	16	25	13	0

Table 2. Nephrectomy [NX] in metastatic RCC: size versus survival (from [5])

	< 10 cm ($n = 48$)		> 10 cm ($n = 52$)	
	NX + %	NX – %	NX + %	NX – %
1 year	52	30	28	26
3 years	30	15	11	0
5 years	25	8	11	0

survival following nephrectomy, no randomized trial that addresses this issue has been reported, and therefore no definitive conclusion can be drawn on this issue.

Spontaneous Regression

Spontaneous regression of metastatic deposits in renal cell carcinoma have been reported in more than 50 cases. In general, these responses have been short lived, limited to minimal pulmonary lesions, and often seen despite simultaneous progression at other sites. In older series the operative mortality of radical nephrectomy in the face of metastatic disease performed in an effort to induce spontaneous regression ranged from 2% to 15%. Montie et al. summarized the reported literature by concluding that less than 1% of patients treated with radical nephrectomy show evidence of spontaneous regression [3]. The evidence thus suggests that this approach is not justifiable.

Solitary Metastases

Combined surgical approaches including excision of solitary or minimal volume metastases and concomitant radical nephrectomy is appropriate in selected patients. These are generally patients with pulmonary, bony, or brain metastases with a good performance status, in whom resection of the metastases does not result in a significant functional deficit in the patient's day-to-day activities. Several studies have documented 5-year survival rates in the order of 25%–35% using this approach for solitary or limited volume metastases in the lung, bones, brain, retroperitoneum, and other sites [6–9]. Unfortunately, most patients treated by this approach with synchronous or metachronous solitary metastases are not cured surgically. Given the relatively low rates of cure even with currently available immunotherapy regimens and prolonged 5-year survival in patients so treated, radical nephrectomy with excision of solitary metastases seems justified. Patients who later fail at other sites would then be candidates for systemic therapy.

Palliative Nephrectomy

The indications for palliative radical nephrectomy include pain, persistent and significant gross hematuria with or without anemia, Budd-Chiari syndrome, hypercalcemia refractory to medical management, cardiac failure owing to intratumoral arteriovenous shunting, and other paraneoplastic syndromes. These symptoms occur only rarely with sufficient severity to justify operation. Montie et al. reported that 32 of 78 patients (41%) with metastatic renal cell carcinoma had no local symptoms prior to death, and that only 17% required nephrectomy for the purpose of palliation of local symptoms [3]. Since patients who present with metastatic renal cancer face an overall survival of short duration, palliative nephrectomy should be restricted to those patients who cannot be managed by nonoperative therapy. Angioinfarction by radiographic embolization of the renal artery may be an equally effective method of managing many of these symptoms. Hypercalcemia and paraneoplastic syndromes can also arise from hormones secreted by metastatic deposits which would not be affected by nephrectomy.

Tumor-Infiltrating Lymphocytes

The role of TILs in treating metastatic disease is now well established. In most instances, the primary tumor serves as the source of TILs. These cells contain both antigen-specific and -nonspecific cytotoxic lymphocytes. Preclinical studies have demonstrated that interleukin-2 activated TILs are 50–100 times more potent than lymphokine-activated killer cells, and that when used clinically, significant antitumor responses occur in metastatic renal tumors [10]. Laboratory methods for harvesting therapeutic doses of TILs ranging from 10^9 to 10^{11} cells per infusion are also well established [10]. While overall response rates to therapy have varied among institutions, this approach is worthy of continued study, and nephrectomy to harvest TILs remains a reasonable approach.

Improving Response to Immunotherapy

The role of radical nephrectomy prior to the administration of systemic immunotherapy is very controversial. Theoretically, radical nephrectomy would debulk the volume of tumor present and thereby decrease the therapeutic burden on the immune system. Nephrectomy might also eliminate trapping of antitumor lymphocytes which would otherwise be diverted from attacking metastatic deposits. At present there is little experimental support for either of these concepts. Belldegrun et al. have reported that patients treated with high-dose systemic interferon-alpha who had undergone preimmunotherapy nephrectomy showed a combined complete and partial response rate of 24% versus 8% in nonnephrectomized patients matched for performance status and volume of pulmonary metastases [11]. The major disadvantage of preimmunotherapy nephrectomy is the potential morbidity of this procedure in patients who may not have optimal performance status. Another disadvantage is that a significant proportion of patients (20% in our experience and 37% in the NCI series) may be prevented from receiving potentially curative therapy because of intercurrent tumor progression, operative complications, or insufficient renal function [12]. The ultimate role of this approach must await the results of randomized trials using standard immunotherapy regimens which match patients for volume of disease.

Postimmunotherapy Nephrectomy

The advantage of postponing radical nephrectomy until after treatment with systemic immunotherapy includes the avoidance of a major surgical procedure and not missing the opportunity for potentially curative systemic therapy. On a theoretical basis, an in situ kidney may serve as a continuing source of tumor antigens which can continue to recruit new antitumor lymphocytes. Fleischman and Kim reported on nine patients treated in this manner [13]. Of three patients who had systemic complete responses to interleukin-2 (IL-2), two were rendered surgically free of disease by posttherapy radical nephrectomy. Both tumor specimens contained less than 1% viable tumor. More recently, Spencer et al. reported on a series of 12 patients treated with IL-2 and interferon-alpha who underwent posttherapy nephrectomy 28–107 days following treatment [14]. All of these patients had excellent performance status and a relatively young mean age (57 years). Patients were treated with one cycle of immunotherapy followed

Table 3. Postimmunotherapy nephrectomy in metastatic RCC: response to interleukin-2 (IL-2) and interferon-alpha (IFN-α)

	Complete response	Partial response	No response/ progressive disease
After 1 cycle IL-2/IFN-α			
Primary tumor[a]	0	0	12
Systemic[b]	1	2	9
After IL-2/IFN-α and nephrectomy	1[c]	0	11

[a] All had histologically viable tumor.
[b] Responses in lung only.
[c] At 11+ months.

by radical nephrectomy. There were four adjunctive procedures including colectomy, partial hepatectomy, and excision of a retroperitoneal mass. Morbidity in these patients was insignificant, and the mean hospital stay was 8.5 days. No clinical or pathological response was seen in the primary tumor of any patient, and all patients had histologically viable tumor upon pathological sectioning (Table 3). Only three patients had responses at extrarenal sites, which were limited to pulmonary metastases. Overall only one patient had a complete response (of 11+ months duration) after treatment with one cycle of IL-2, interferon-alpha, and radical nephrectomy. The remaining 11 patients all had progressive disease at the time of last follow-up. While this approach seems feasible with minimal morbidity and may carry some advantages over pre-immunotherapy nephrectomy, its overall value has not yet been proven, and further studies are required to refine its role.

Summary and Conclusions

The role of radical nephrectomy in the management of metastatic renal cell carcinoma continues to evolve as our understanding of the interaction between renal cell carcinoma and the immune system expands. At present it appears reasonable and justifiable to perform radical nephrectomy in the face of metastatic disease in the following situations: (a) with concomitant excision of solitary or low-volume metastases; (b) for harvesting TILs; and (c) rarely for palliation of local or systemic symptoms which cannot be managed non-operatively. It appears unjustifiable to perform radical nephrectomy in the hope of induction of spontaneous regression of metastases.

Finally, more study is needed on the impact of nephrectomy on the host immune response either before or after systemic immunotherapy. There are several unanswered questions in regard to these issues. For example, it is not yet clear that pretherapy nephrectomy indeed enhances the response to immunotherapy. If this is borne out by randomized studies, it will be important to understand whether and why the same effect can be achieved by other, perhaps nonsurgical means. It is also not clear whether adjunctive nephrectomy will work equally well with all forms of immunotherapy. The impact of tumor size and metastatic burden must be controlled for in new studies, and the morbidity of preimmunotherapy nephrectomy which denies potentially curative therapy to approximately 30% of patients must be examined more closely.

The approach of postimmunotherapy nephrectomy also needs more scrutiny. In particular, it is unclear whether extrarenal sites will predictably respond to immunotherapy with the kidney left in situ. The best timing for postimmunotherapy nephrectomy is also unclear, as is whether nephrectomy should be performed after immunotherapy if no systemic response is seen, or only if there is a complete response at all extrarenal sites. Finally, responses in the primary tumor when the kidney is left in situ are rare, and new approaches must be developed to induce regression at the primary site in a higher proportion of patients.

References

1. Johnson DE, Kaesler KE, Samuels ML (1975) Is nephrectomy justified in patients with metastatic renal cell carcinoma. J Urol 114: 27
2. Klugo RC, Detmers M, Stiles RE et al. (1977) Aggressive versus conservative management of stage IV renal cell carcinoma. J Urol 118: 244
3. Montie JE, Stewart BH, Straffon RA et al. (1977) The role of adjunctive nephrectomy in patients with metastatic renal cell carcinoma. J Urol 117: 272
4. Patel NP, Lavengood RW (1978) Renal cell carcinoma: natural history and results of treatment. J Urol 119: 722
5. Frank J (1992) Nephrectomy in metastatic renal cell carcinoma. J Urol 147: 421A
6. Tolia BM, Whitmore WF (1975) Solitary metastases from renal cell carcinoma. J Urol 114: 836
7. Middleton RG (1967) Surgery for metastatic renal cell carcinoma. J Urol 97: 973
8. deKernion JB, Ramming KD, Smith RB (1978) The natural history of metastatic renal cell carcinoma: a computer analysis. J Urol 120: 148
9. O'Dea MJ, Zincke H, Utz DC et al. (1978) The treatment of renal cell carcinoma with solitary metastases. J Urol 120: 540
10. Bukowski R, Murthy S, Klein EA et al. Tumor infiltrating lymphocytes in metastatic renal cell carcinoma: the Cleveland clinic experience. In: Klein EA, Bukowski R, Finke J (eds) The immunobiology of renal cell carcinoma. (in press)
11. Belldegrun A, Webb DE, Austin HA et al. (1989) Renal toxicity of interleukin-II administration in patients with metastatic renal cell cancer: effect of pretherapy nephrectomy. J Urol 141: 499
12. Robertson CN, Linehan WM, Pass HI et al. (1990) Preparative cytoreductive surgery in patients with metastatic renal cell carcinoma, treated with adoptive immunotherapy with interleukin-II or interleukin-II plus lymphokine-activated killer cells. J Urol 144: 614

13. Fleischmann J, Kim B (1991) Interleukin-2 immunotherapy followed by resection of residual renal cell carcinoma. J Urol 145: 938
14. Spencer WF, Linehan WM, Walther MM et al. (1992) Immunotherapy with IL-2 and alpha interferon in patients with metastatic renal cell cancer with in situ primary cancers: a pilot study. J Urol 147: 24
15. Fowler JE (1987) Urol Clin North Am 14: 745–756

Possibilities and Limitations of Surgery for Liver Metastases of Renal Cell Cancer

P. Hohenberger

Incidence of Liver Metastases in Renal Cell Carcinoma

The experience with any surgical treatment for liver metastases of renal cell carcinoma is very limited. This may be due to the distribution of distant metastases to different organs. Considering first the results of autopsy studies, the data collected by Pickren et al. [24] suggest that substantial attention has been attracted to the liver as a site of metastases. About 40% of patients present with these at death; 33% presented no liver metastases, and 27% presented no distant metastases. An incidence of about 40% is confirmed by other autopsy studies [9], indicating that liver metastases are less common than lung metastases (72%) but more common than, for example, brain metastases (22%). Considering the distribution of metastases (Table 1), patients with isolated liver metastases are exceptional, and these authors observe that the more organs are involved, the higher the incidence of liver deposits [9, 28].

These facts reflect the clinical situation. Even authors with a special interest in the treatment of metastatic renal cell carcinoma rarely if ever treat patients with liver metastases [34]. In a series of patients with metastatic renal cell carcinoma evaluated prospectively for survival only 11% had liver metastases [7]. Reports focusing on the surgical treatment of renal cell carcinoma with solitary metastases have not included patients with liver metastases [8, 21]; this was also the case in a series reporting on an aggressive treatment policy in renal cell carcinoma [12].

Considerations of the Anatomy of Liver Metastases as a Prerequisite for Liver Resection

The metastatic behavior of renal cell carcinoma does not favor surgical treatment. In contrast to colon cancer, with its portal venous route of hematogenous metastases making the liver the first organ filter, renal cell cancer shows a caval type of dissemination, and the liver represents only one organ involved in the

Chirurgische Universitätsklinik, Im Neuenheimer Feld 110, D-69120 Heidelberg, Germany

Table 1. Distribution of liver metastases to different organs in autopsy studies of patients who died from renal cell cancer

	Lungs %	Brain %	Liver %
Number of organs			
One	71	17	0, 5[a]
Two	77	27	38, 25[a]
Three	64	33	56
Four	100	46	54
Overall	72	22	48

[a] Data from Saitoh et al. [28].

metastatic process. Furthermore, little is known about the anatomical peculiarities of liver deposits of hypernephroma that would provide a basis for resection. These prerequisites derived from liver resection in colorectal cancer are: unidirectional drainage of tumor cells to the liver, small margin of angiogenesis and neovascularisation (about 3–5 mm), noninfiltrative growth (invasion of major branches of the intrahepatic portal vein is rare), and an invasional area of only 5–10 cell layers of liver cells to enable resections with clear margins of 1–2 cm. In renal cell carcinoma such systemic examinations on the anatomical details of liver metastases must still be performed to make liver resection with curative intent a reasonable procedure.

Experience and Results of Liver Resection in Renal Cell Carcinoma

Liver resection for renal cell carcinoma metastases has a rare indication. Of 13 series published reporting results of resection of liver metastases for various primary tumors only 2.2% of the operative procedures had been performed for renal cell carcinoma. This survey (Table 2) encompasses 39 resections, but in some reports it is not clear whether resections were performed for Wilms' tumors or for renal cell cancers [25]. Additionally, only seven authors report on their treatment results, and only four patients surviving for 5 years or more are documented.

Experience and Results of Intra-arterial Chemo-/Immunotherapy in Renal Cell Carcinoma

Patients with liver metastases of renal cell cancer could be candidates for regional intrahepatic chemotherapy. Again, few experiences have been reported in the literature. Some patients have been treated by doxorubicin [17, 18].

Table 2. Studies of liver resection for metastases in renal cell cancer

Reference	Number of resections	Number of survivors at (years)
Ramming et al. [25]	8/123	Two at 5 years
Foster and Lundy [10]	5/335	Two at 2 years
Morrow et al. [20]	1/ 64	ND
Thompson et al. [36]	1/138	One at 5 years
Tomas-de la Vega et al. [37]	3/ 29	Two at 5 years
Kortz et al. [16]	1/ 21	ND
Funovics et al. [11]	4/245	ND
Ringe et al. [26]	5/151	ND
Stimpson et al. [32]	1/ 87	ND
Cobourn et al. [4]	1/ 56	ND
Iwatsuki and Starzl [14]	3/411	None at 5 years
Stehlin et al. [30]	4/111	One at 5 years
Sturm et al. [33]	2/ 34	One at 5 years
Total	39/1805 (2.2%)	

ND, No data available on follow-up.

Partial responses were reported in two patients, and another patient subsequently underwent lobectomy of the right hepatic lobe [18]. Another chemotherapeutic regimen included 5-fluoro-2-deoxyuridine-c8 (with two partial responses in four patients) [38]. Treatment using mitomycin combined with 5-fluorouracil resulted in progressive disease in three patients [30]. Taniguchi et al. used ethiodized oil (Lipiodol) in combination with multiple cytostatic drugs. As the oil is retained by liver tumors, the uptake of drugs should be improved by continuous release from the suspension [35]; control of metastatic growth was reported, but no detailed data on the type of tumors were given.

We treated a 45-year-old man with continuous alpha-interferon (10×10^6 U daily for 5 days) via the hepatic artery. Six months of stable disease had been observed before he died after another 2 months from rapidly growing lung metastases.

Recently, approaches with regional immunotherapy for liver tumors have been described. Codde et al. reported on animal experiments using intra-arterial gamma-interferon that demonstrate increased efficacy compared to systemic application [5]. Mavligit et al. used rhTNF administered continuously in patients with liver metastases from melanoma, colorectal, and breast cancer. The response rate to treatment was 14%, with severe hypophosphatemia and myocardial ischemia complicating this schedule [19]. Improved efficacy of regional interleukin-2 has been demonstrated following administration to the splenic artery for liver metastases of malignant melanoma [15]. The overall response rate in 43 patients treated was 29%, including two complete remissions.

Other Approaches to the Treatment of Liver Metastases in Renal Cell Carcinoma

Recently some new approaches to the nonresectional treatment of liver tumors have been reported. Mainly patients with colorectal metastases have been treated, but also patients with metastases of different primary tumors including those of renal cell cancer have been investigated.

Cryosurgical destruction of liver metastases guided by ultrasonography is one of these efforts. Metastases and a small rim of liver tissue are frozen for 15–180 min at $-180°C$, and alterations in the lesion are monitored by ultrasound [2]. Tumor types treated up to now include leiomyosarcoma and colorectal, and carcinoid metastases. Treatment mortality, however, has been 5.6%, and major hemorrhage, renal failure, and injuries to the bile ducts have been reported.

Isolated hyperthermic liver perfusion is another approach. This procedure was developed in 1961 [3] and has been applied in a larger series of patients by Aigner [1]. This enables chemotherapeutic agents to be added to the perfusion circuit in doses higher than would be tolerated by systemic administration. Treatment is complicated by intractable bleedings from metastases and septicemia. Control of hepatic metastases is not always achieved, and additional chemotherapy via the hepatic artery is recommended. Today this procedure is used almost exclusively in animal experiments to evaluate the effects of high-dose regional chemotherapy of new drugs.

Embolization has rarely been applied for the treatment of renal cell cancer metastatic to the liver. Coldwell and Mortimer reported on three patients with hypervascular lesions treated with injection of polyvinyl alcohol foam (Ivalon) to the hepatic artery until vascular stasis occurred [6]. While tumor regression was observed in colorectal and carcinoid metastases, only one patient with renal cell cancer metastases developed a minor response. However, liver tumors derive their blood supply from different areas after occlusion of the hepatic artery (diaphragm, minor omentum); therefore other treatment modalities are under consideration.

To avoid the development of collateral circulation intermittent desarterialization has been proposed. The combination of sequential ischemia and intra-arterial chemotherapy can be administered by use of a vascular occluder (balloon catheter) operatively sewn around the hepatic artery and connected to a subcutaneous port. Injection of saline to the port leads to a temporary occlusion. A daily period of ischemia of 1–2 h is followed by 5-fluorouracil via the hepatic artery. The rationale of this treatment is based on synchronization of the cell cycle in tumor tissue after release of circulation, making the subsequent infusion of cytotoxic drugs more effective. Initial observations in patients have shown calcifications occurring within the metastases and the median survival of patients with colorectal metastases to be slightly better than those after intra-arterial chemotherapy alone [23].

Relevance of Surgery for Immunotherapy

Experience with liver resection and regional surgical treatment modalities is very limited in renal cell cancer. However, it is necessary to anticipate interactions of surgery and immunotherapy if surgical efforts are to be a prerequisite for immunotherapy, for example, debulking procedures or for harvesting of tumor-infiltrating lymphocytes. This means discussing morbidity, immunological alterations, and the influence on metastatic growth induced by surgery.

Morbidity and Mortality of Liver Resection

The morbidity associated with liver resection in renal cell cancer depends upon the treatment of metastatic colorectal cancer. Operative mortality is reported to be less than 10% in larger series [13, 14, 26]. A total of 182 patients underwent liver resection for colorectal metastases between 1981 and 1991 in our Department. Deaths occurred only in cases of right hemihepatectomy ($n = 3$) and extended right hemihepatectomy ($n = 2$) leaving behind only segments 1–3 of the left liver lobe. Minor resections such as segmentectomies, bisegmentectomies, and left hemihepatectomies were performed in 99 patients without hospital mortality (Table 3).

Reports on morbidity and mortality in resection of noncolorectal metastases, including those of renal cell cancer, are rare. Ramming et al. [25] and Stehlin et al. [30] are the only authors who have reported on mortality in these patients, which seems acceptable for the treatment of metastatic disease (Table 3).

Table 3. Morbidity and mortality in liver resection for metastatic disease

	Morbidity %	Mortality %
Colorectal metastases		
Own experience, all patients ($n = 182$)	24	3.2
Own experience, hemihepatectomies ($n = 84$)	38	6.6
Own experience, segmental resections ($n = 98$)	12	0
Noncolorectal metastases		
Ramming et al. [25] ($n = 40$)	46	10.5
Iwatsuki and Starzl [14] ($n = 33$)		0
Stehlin et al. [30] ($n = 68$)	32	6.5
Own experience ($n = 15$)	20	0

Morbidity data include pneumonia, pleural effusion, subphrenic abscesses, wound or urinary tract infection, sepsis, hepatic failure, and cardiac events.

Immunomodulatory Effects of Liver Resection

The rate of complications after liver resection appears proportional to blood loss [32]. Younes et al. evaluated the influence of blood transfusions on survival in patients undergoing liver resection for colorectal metastases at the Memorial Sloan Kettering Cancer Center [39]. While the transfusion of packed red cells had no influence on survival, whole-blood transfusions adversely effected treatment results. Similar data reported Stephenson et al. who analyzed the data on 59 patients undergoing resection of isolated hepatic metastases at the NCI [31]. Both overall survival and period free of recurrence were decreased in patients who had received blood transfusions perioperatively. Avoidance of blood transfusions is therefore of major interest during liver resection for secondary cancer. This can be afforded by careful selection of patients, sophisticated operative technique, and the use of transfusion of autologous blood only. In a series of patients treated in that way, Ryan and Faulkner reported a transfusion rate of 6% in their patients [27]. In our experience with a similar policy as that described above, only 11% of 65 patients undergoing liver resections during the past 2 years required transfusion of heterologous blood components.

Besides transfusion, intraoperative hypotension is thought to be a factor in decreased survival postoperatively [32]. Younes and coworkers carefully evaluated anesthesia charts and disease-free survival following resection of colorectal liver for cure [39]. Hypotension was defined as a decrease in mean arterial pressure to less than 80% of baseline. Patients with more than three episodes lasting more than 30 min had a significantly shorter disease-free survival in a multivariate analysis ($p = 0.00017$). Cofactors were the site of primary tumor, carcinoembryonic antigen levels, and the number of metastases removed.

Blood loss and hypovolemic shock have been shown significantly to affect the immune system. These events depress mitogen-induced lymphocyte proliferation and the production of interleukin-2 [39]. Therefore it is necessary to avoid these events as they may override positive effects of the resection.

Animal Experiments on Metastases to the Regenerating Liver

One mechanism by which immunosuppression is thought to influence tumor growth is via the activation of micrometastases or dormant tumor cells and by facilitating metastatic growth in the regenerating liver. Several experimental attempts advocating this thesis have been made in immunocompetent animals. Recently, Panis et al. selected animals without overt liver metastases 8 weeks after inoculation of tumor cells to the hepatic artery (autochthonous DMH-induced colon cancer). Subsequently they assigned these animals to either 70% liver resection, treatment with cyclosporin A, or to the control group. After liver resection 62% of the animals developed overt liver metastases, in contrast to 20% in the control group; however, 80% of the animals in the cyclosporin showed growth of metastatic tumor [22]. In another experiment using immuno-(T-cell-)deficient BALB/c mice transplanted with a human colon cancer cell line the effect of liver regeneration on tumor growth kinetics was studied [29]. Inoculation was carried out simultaneously with a 60% liver resection and 1 day, 2 weeks, and 4 weeks after the operation. The simultaneous injection led to metastases in 90% of the animals and the average number of tumor deposits was highest. The longer the period between operation and inoculation of tumor cells, the lower the number and number of metastases was. Both experiments may support the thesis of augmented tumor growth of dormant cells after liver resection irrespective of whether animals were immunocompromized or not.

Conclusions

The metastatic behavior of renal cell cancer does not generally meet the prerequisites for the treatment of liver metastases. In only rare cases is the liver the only location of tumor spread. Furthermore, the anatomical criteria for liver resection (angiogenesis, margin of infiltration, invasion of major branches of the portal vein) are still to be investigated. Therefore the clinical experience with resectional treatment and regional cytostatic chemotherapy is very limited. New regional approaches (cryosurgery, regional immunotherapy, chemoembolization) must still be evaluated in renal cell cancer. Mortality and morbidity of liver resection would be acceptable if treatment of colorectal metastases as a standard is taken as the model. However, immunomodulatory effects of liver resection (blood transfusion, hypotension) may counterbalance the effects of debulking.

References

1. Aigner KR (1988) Isolated liver perfusion: 5-year results. Reg Cancer Treat 1: 11–20
2. Atkinson D, Zemel R, Weaver ML, Onik G (1992) Hepatic cryosurgery for metastatic carcinoma (abstract). Proc ASCO 11: 165
3. Ausman RK (1961) Development of a technique for isolated perfusion of the liver. NY State J Med 61: 3993–3997
4. Cobourn CS, Makowka L, Langer B, Taylor BR, Falk RE (1987) Examination of patients selection and outcome for hepatic resection for metastatic disease. Surg Gynecol Obstet 165: 239–246
5. Codde JP, Vines JA, Burton MA, Gray BN, van der Meide PH (1990) Enhanced efficacy by regional administration of interferon gamma in the treatment of liver tumors. Reg Cancer Treat 3: 163–165
6. Coldwell DM, Mortimer JE (1991) Hepatic artery embolization in the treatment of hepatic malignancies. Reg Cancer Treat 3: 298–301
7. de Kernion JB, Ramming KP, Smith RB (1978) The natural history of metastatic renal cell carcinoma: a computer analysis. J Urol 120: 148–152
8. Dineen MK, Pastore R, Emrich L, Huben RP (1988) Results of surgical treatment of renal cell carcinoma with solitary metastases. J Urol 140: 277–279

9. Eder M (1984) Die Metastasierung: Fakten und Probleme aus humanpathologischer Sicht Verh Dtsch Ges Pathol 68: 1–11
10. Foster JH, Lundy J (1981) Pathology of liver metastasis. Curr Prob Surg 18: 157–164
11. Funovics JM, Wenzl E, Függer R, Schemper M (1986) Leberresektionen wegen hämatogener oder infiltrierender Mestastasen. Wien Klin Wochenschr 98: 813–820
12. Golimbu M, Al-Askari S, Tessler A, Morales P (1986) Aggressive treatment of metastatic renal cell cancer. J Urol 136: 805–808
13. Hohenberger P, Schlag P, Herfarth C (1988) Leberresektion bei Patienten mit Metastasen kolorektaler Karzinome. Chirurg 59: 410–417
14. Iwatsuki S, Starzl T (1989) Personal experience with 411 hepatic resections. Ann Surg 208: 421–434
15. Keilholz U, Schlag P, Tilgen W et al. (1992) Regional administration of lymphokine-activated killer cells can be superior to intravenous application. Cancer 69: 2172–2175
16. Kortz WJ, Myers WC, Hanks JB, Schirmer B, Jones S (1984) Hepatic resection for metastatic cancer. Ann Surg 199: 182–184
17. Kraybill WG, Harrison M, Sasaki T, Fletcher WS (1977) Regional intraarterial infusion of adriamycin in the treatment of cancer. Surg Gynecol Obstet 144: 335–338
18. Kuwamitsu O, Kubota Y, Miura T, Shuin T, Hosaka M, Sugiyama K (1990) Intraarterial chemotherapy combined with surgery for liver metastasis of renal cell carcinoma. Reg Cancer Treat 3: 166–168
19. Mavligit G, Zukiwski A, Charnsangavej C, Carrasco CH, Wallace S, Gutterman JU (1992) Regional biologic therapy. Hepatic arterial infusion of recombinant human tumor necrosis factor in patients with liver metastases. Cancer 69: 557–561
20. Morrow CE, Grage TB, Sutherland DER, Najarian JS (1982) Hepatic resection for secondary neoplasms. Surgery 92: 610–614
21. O'Dea MJ, Zincke H, Utz D, Bernatz PE (1978) The treatment of renal cell carcinoma with solitary metastasis. J Urol 120: 540–543
22. Panis Y, Ribeiro J, Chretien Y, Nordlinger B (1992) Dormat liver metastases: an experimental study. Br J Surg 79: 221–223
23. Persson B, Jeppson B, Ekberg H, Tranberg KG, Lundstedt C, Bengmark S (1990) Repeated dearterialization of hepatic tumors with an implantable occluder. Cancer 66: 1139–1146
24. Pickren JW, Tsukada Y, Lane W (1984) Liver metastases: analysis of autopsy data. In: Weiss L, Gilber HA (eds) Liver metastases. Hall, Boston, pp 2–18
25. Ramming KP, Sparks FC, Eilber F, Morton D (1977) Management of hepatic metastases. Semin Oncol 4: 71–80
26. Ringe B, Bechstein WO, Raab R, Meyer HJ, Pichlmayr R (1990) Leberresektion bei 157 Patienten mit colorectalen Metastasen. Chirurg 61: 272–279
27. Ryan JA, Faulkner DJ (1989) Liver resection without blood transfusion. Am J Surg 157: 472–475
28. Saitoh H, Hida M, Nakamura K, Shimbo T, Shiramizu T, Satoh T (1982) Metastatic processes and a potential indication of treatment for metastatic lesions of renal adenocarcinoma. J Urol 128: 916–918
29. Schackert K, Price J, Avallone A, Fidler IJ (1992) Influence of liver regeneration on the biological behaviour of human tumor metastases in athymic nude mice. In: Hartel W, Beger HG, Ungeheuar E (eds) Archiv für Chirurgie. Supplement. Chirurgisches Forum 191 für experimentelle und Klinische Forschung, Springer, Berlin Heidelberg New York, pp 21–26
30. Stehlin J, de Ipolyi P, Greeff P, McGraff CJ, Davis B, McNary L (1988) Treatment of cancer of the liver. Twenty years experience with infusion and resection in 414 patients. Ann Surg 208: 23–35
31. Stephenson KR, Steinberg S, Hughes KS, Vetto JT, Sugarbaker Ph, Chang AE (1988) Perioperative blood transfusions are associated with decreased time to recurrence

and decreased survival after resection of isolated colorectal liver metastases. Ann Surg 208: 679–687
32. Stimpson RE, Pellegrini CA, Way LW (1987) Factors affecting the morbidity of elective liver resection. Am J Surg 153: 189–196
33. Sturm J, Raute M, Trede M (1991) Perationsindikation bei Lebermetastasen nicht-kolorektaler Karzinome. In: Herfarth C, Schlag P (eds) Neue Entwicklungen in Therapie von Lebertumoren. Springer, Berlin Heidelberg New York, pp 337–344
34. Swanson DA, Johnson DE, von Eschenbach A, Chuang VP, Wallace S (1983) Angioinfarction plus nephrectomy for metastaic renal cell carcinoma – an update. J Urol 130: 4498–452
35. Taniguchi R, Takahashi T, Yamaguchi T, Sawai K (1989) Intraarterial infusion chemotherapy for metastatic liver tumors using multiple anti-cancer agents suspended in a lipid contrast medium. Cancer 64: 2001–2006
36. Thompson H, Tompkins R, Longmire WP (1983) Major hepatic resection. Ann Surg 197: 375–388
37. Tomas-de la Vega JE, Donahue EJ, Doolas A (1984) A ten years experience with hepatic resection. Surg Gynecol Obstet 159: 223–228
38. Yamashita Y, Takahashi M, Bussaka H, Fukushima S, Kawaguchi T, Nakano M (1989) Intraarterial infusion of 5-fluoro-2-deoxyuridine-c8 dissolved in a lymphographic agent in malignant liver tumors. Cancer 64: 2437–2444
39. Younes R, Rogatko R, Brennan MF (1991) The influence of intraoperative hypotension and perioperative transfusion on disease-free survival in patients with complete resection of colorectal liver metastases. Ann Surg 214: 107–113

The Role of Bone Surgery for Immunotherapy in Disseminated Renal Cell Cancer

W. Friedl and T. Fritz

Hypernephroma is one of the five tumors with the highest incidence of metastases and pathological fractures. The high incidence of pathological fractures in hypernephroma as compared with that in prostate carcinoma, which has an even higher incidence of bone metastases, is due to the osteolytic type of metastasis in hypernephroma versus the osteoplastic type in prostate cancer.

Up to 1982 breast cancer was responsible for about two-thirds of all pathological fractures in our hospital. In recent years, however, hypernephroma was the most frequent tumor causing pathological fractures [2]. Many factors probably contribute to this change. The wide use of osteoclast-inactivating diphosphonates (Ostac) in patients with breast cancer has significantly decreased the number of pathological fractures in breast cancer patients [8]. On the other hand, the development of many new procedures for operative stabilization of pathological fractures and the knowledge of these possibilities has significantly increased the number of patients in our institution presenting with pathological or impending pathological fractures with other primary carcinomas. Surgical management of bone metastases in patients with RCC is indicated when the quality of life can be improved by surgical management [7]. This is true in pathological or impending pathological fractures or when large tumor masses cause local mechanical problems or skin ulceration. By metastasis resection and stabilization of the skeleton the condition of the patient can be improved so that other therapy modalities such as immunotherapy can be performed. The tumor cells of bone metastasis can be used for active, specific immunization. Bone metastasis resection also contributes to tumor mass reduction and may thus improve the efficacy of immunotherapy. Whereas bone metastases are most frequent in cancellous bone such as the spine because of the higher blood supply, pathological fractures are found more frequently in long bones, especially the proximal femur, because of the higher biomechanical load in this part of the skeleton (Fig. 1).

There are many definitions of impending pathological fractures [6], but the most important criterion for differentiating an impending from a nonimpending pathological fracture is the presence of load- or function-dependent pain. Other

Chirurgische Universitatsklinik, Abteilung Unfallchirurgie, Im Neuenheimer Feld 110, D-69120 Heidelberg, Germany

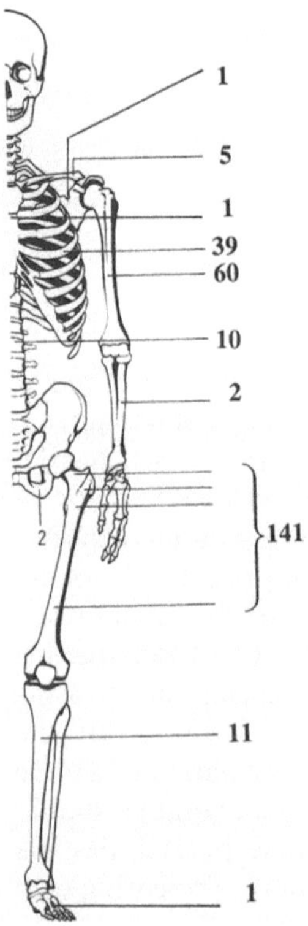

Fig. 1. Distribution of pathological fractures in the skeleton observed 1972–1989

criteria include a metastasis diameter greater than 2.5 cm and destruction of more than 50% of cortical bone in a loaded area of the skeleton. A pathological fracture is not always evident on an X-ray.

The indication for surgical management of pathological fractures depends on many factors; these influence both the primary therapy option and the procedure to be used. They include the following.

Life expectancy of the patient is one of the most important factors. Because the mean life expectancy of patients with pathological fractures is only 5–15 months in different examinations, immediate relief of pain and restoration of function and weight-bearing capacity are necessary. In patients with a life expectancy over 3 months metastasis resection and stabilization should generally be recommended. This avoids progression of local metastasis and thus instability of the osteosynthesis. Intramedullary stabilization without metastasis resection also distributes the tumor cells in the whole medullar space, with the risk of secondary local metastases and tumor cell embolization. Stabilization must also be performed under consideration of the biomechanical stress of the part of the skeleton affected to avoid implant instability and the necessity of second operations (Figs. 2, 3).

Localization of the metastases is also important. The most frequent localization of metastases is in the extremities; surgical management is the first choice

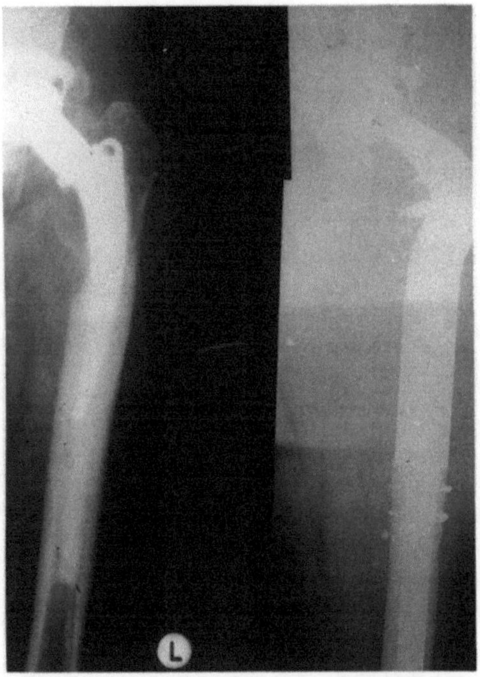

Fig. 2. Local recurrence after non-radical local resection of a femor neck metastasis and postoperative radiotherapy

here because it is now possible to restore immediately the weight-bearing capacity and function in all cases, with very low morbidity and mortality. Pain caused by instability is relieved immediately. This leads to short hospitalization and significant improvement in the patient's quality of life. In spine and pelvis metastasis radiotherapy is used first. When this is not effective, or neurological symptoms occur, surgical management is indicated.

If a pathological fracture has already occurred, surgical management is generally indicated.

In impending pathological fractures of the leg and arm surgical management is the first choice. The best time for surgical management of bone metastases is with the impending pathological fracture. Functional results are best in patients with impending pathological fractures because the patients immediately regain their normal preoperative function. In patients with spine and pelvis metastases radiotherapy may be used first because of the higher morbidity of surgery in these parts of the skeleton. In the case of tumor progression or the occurrence of neurological symptoms surgical stabilization must be performed.

Regarding the number of metastases, operative therapy is indicated in single or singular metastases with pathological or impending pathological fracture. Single metastases are typical for hypernephroma.

The presence of neurological damage and the time from appearance are also important considerations. Operative metastasis resection and stabilization

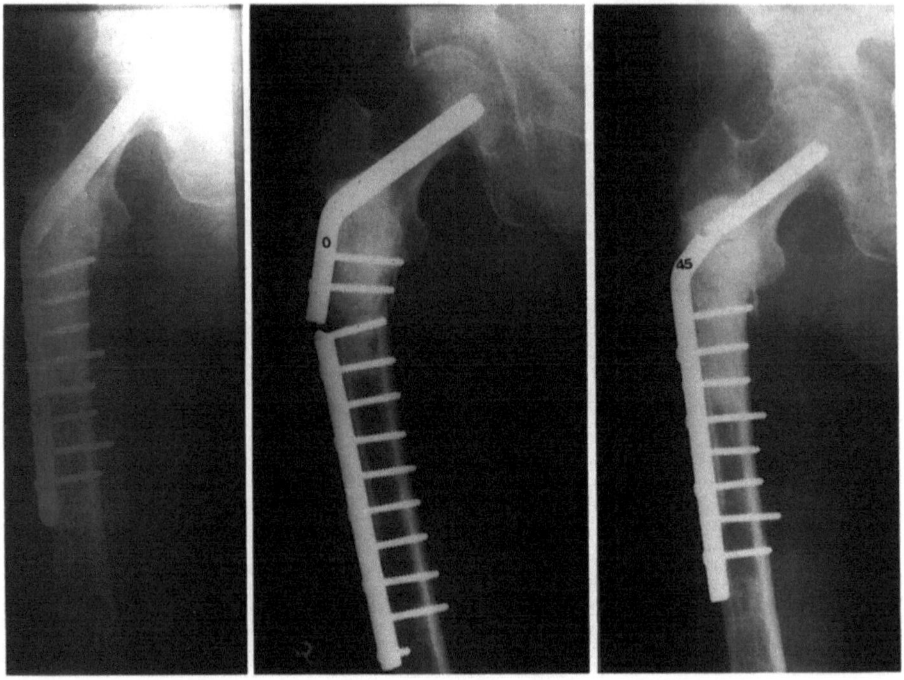

Fig. 3. Instability after intralesional metastasis resection and simple angle plate compound osteosynthesis. Fatigue instability of the plate because of the lacking medial cortical or implant support

should be performed in the first 6 h and not later than 24 h after the appearance of neurological symptoms caused by spinal cord or nerve compression.

Hypernephroma metastases have high vascularity. In very extended metastases or unfavorable anatomical sites in terms of bleeding control, preoperative embolization should be performed. In our opinion, the indication must be restrictive in spine metastases because neurological deficit is reported in 5%–10% after embolization . This is caused by spinal cord ischemia at the level of embolization.

Other factors to be considered include:

surgical resectability of the lesion,
availability of other therapy options,
general condition of the patient, and
experience of the surgeon.

These principles are illustrated below for the most important sites of the skeleton [4].

The proximal femur is the most common site of pathological fractures. When the metastasis is located in the femur head, neck, or the greater trochanter, only resection of the hip joint with the proximal femur and tumor prosthesis

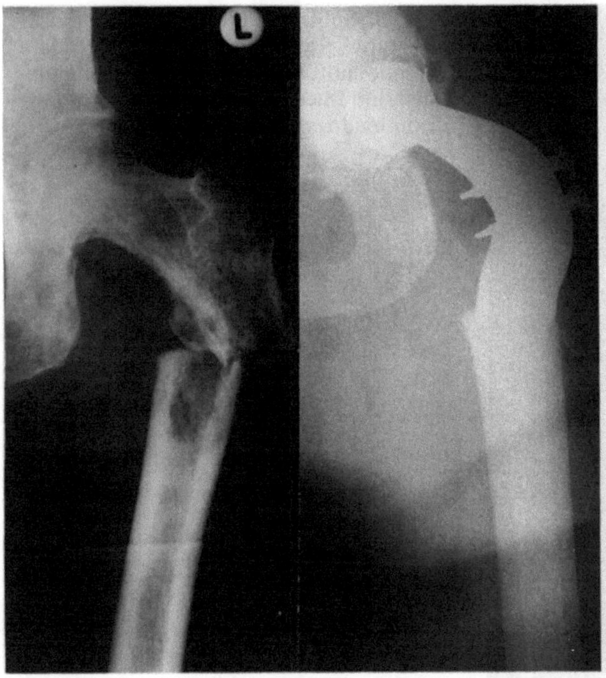

Fig. 4. Intertrochanteric pathological fracture. Therapy with tumor prosthesis

replacement can be performed (Fig. 4). The tumor prosthesis has the disadvantage that the abductor muscles must be inserted on the trunk of the prosthesis. Therefore one often sees luxations of the prosthesis. In all cases in which the metastasis is localized below the intertrochanteric level and down to the supracondylar region, the stabilization can be performed by the procedure we call double plate compound osteosynthesis [5] (Figs. 5, 6). This allows complete resection of the metastasis with the surrounding tissue and in all cases a primary full weight-bearing capacity. Experimental data showed a loading capacity similar to that of non osteotomized normal femora [3]. Clinical use of this device shows that the rate of local complications is much lower compared with tumor prosthesis of the hip. This is caused only by the high luxation rate of the prosthesis. In 30 patients with tumor prosthesis operated on between 1985 and 1989, 11 luxations in 7 patients were observed. A simple hip prosthesis would not entail these problems, but sufficient local control is not possible with such a system even when postoperative radiotherapy is added, as was observed in earlier decades.

When the knee is involved, only individual or modular system knee prostheses can be used. In the tibia we also use double plate compound osteosynthesis systems (Fig. 7).

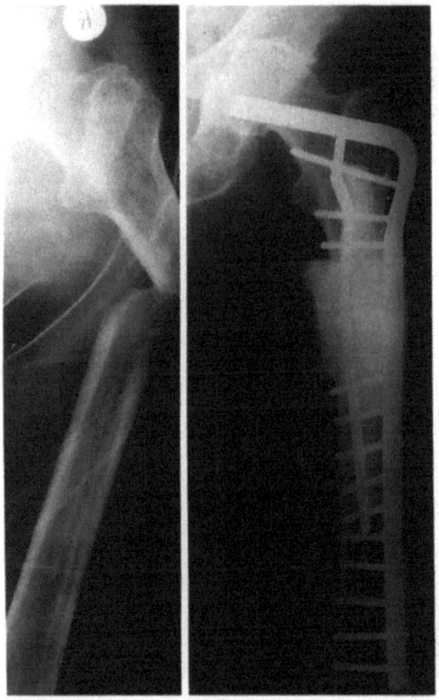

Fig. 5. Subtrochanteric pathological fracture. Resection and double plate compound osteosynthesis. Note the medial intramedullary plate for compression load transmission

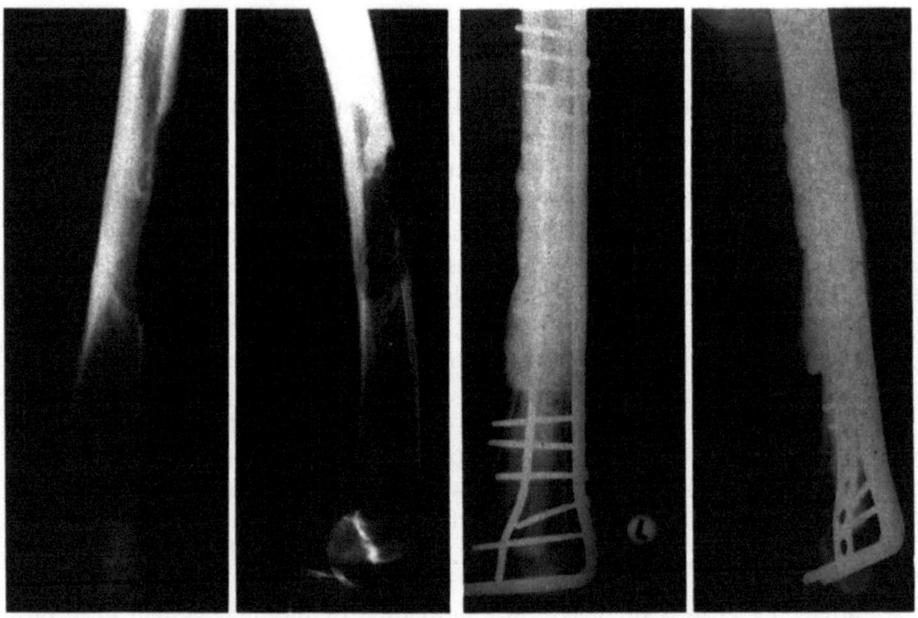

a b

Fig. 6a, b. Reversed double plate compound osteosynthesis in distal femur shaft metastasis and impending pathological fracture

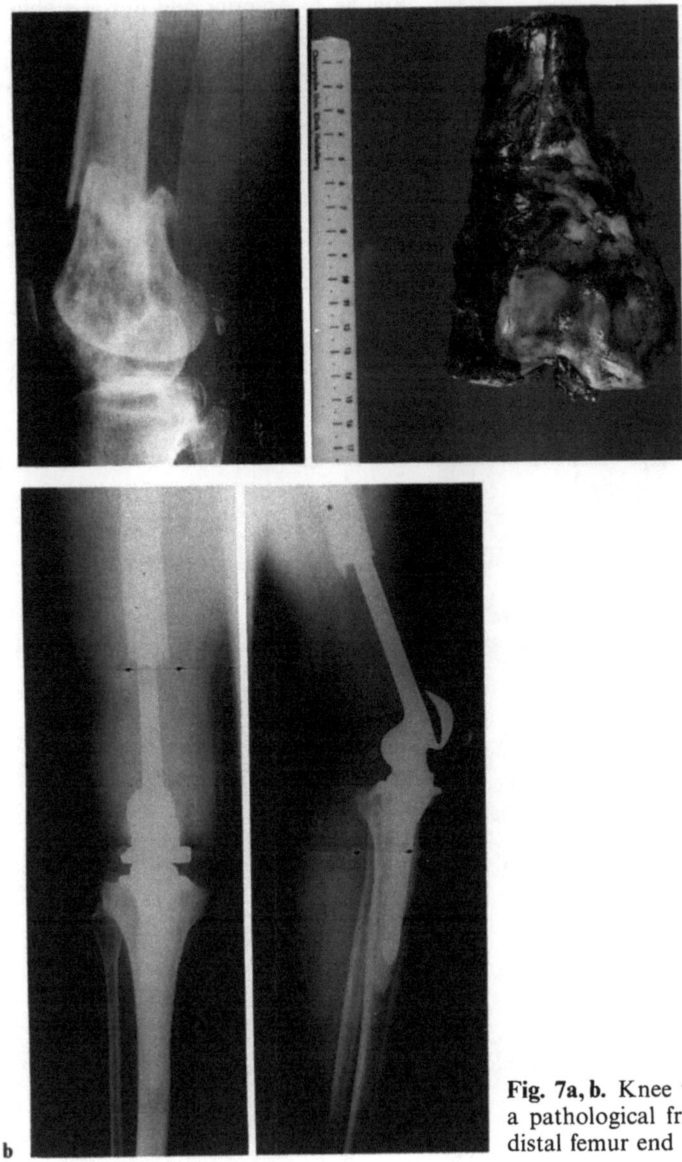

a

b

Fig. 7a, b. Knee tumor prosthesis in a pathological fracture affecting the distal femur end

In patients with very poor general condition and a life expectancy less than 3 months, locking nail systems such as the gamma nail in an intertrochanteric fracture and a locked femur nail in shaft fractures should be used. The Ender nail osteosynthesis should no longer be used because there is no real immobilization of the fracture, and dislocation is very common.

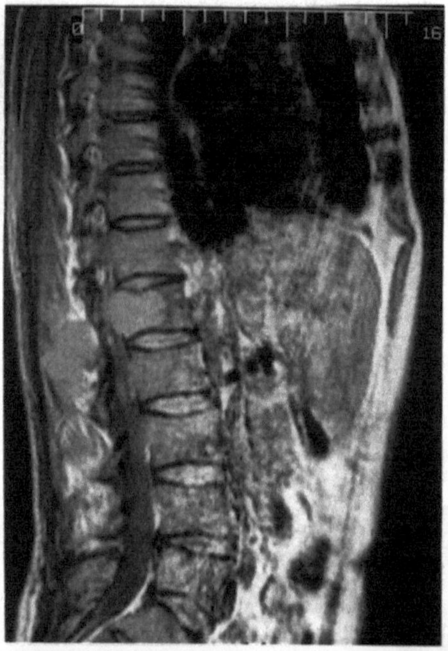

a

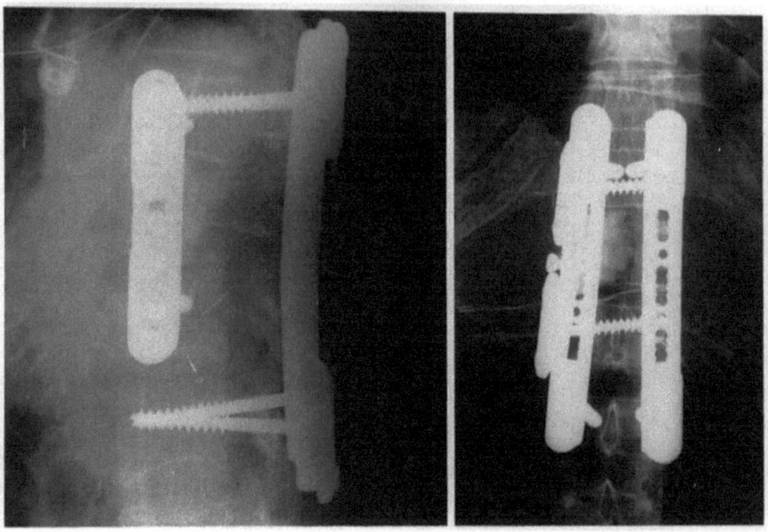

b

Fig. 8a, b. Anterior and dorsal stabilization in a pathological lumbal spine fracture. Preoperative magnetic resonance imaging and postoperative plain X-ray control

In spine metastases in patients with a life expectancy greater than 3–6 months metastasis resection is also necessary. The approach depends on the site of the lesion. Because the ventral parts are generally affected, the vertebral body must be resected. Stabilization is performed by a compound plate fixator osteosynthesis. If the dorsal parts are also affected, combined resection and stabilization must be performed (Fig. 8). Isolated dorsal decompression and

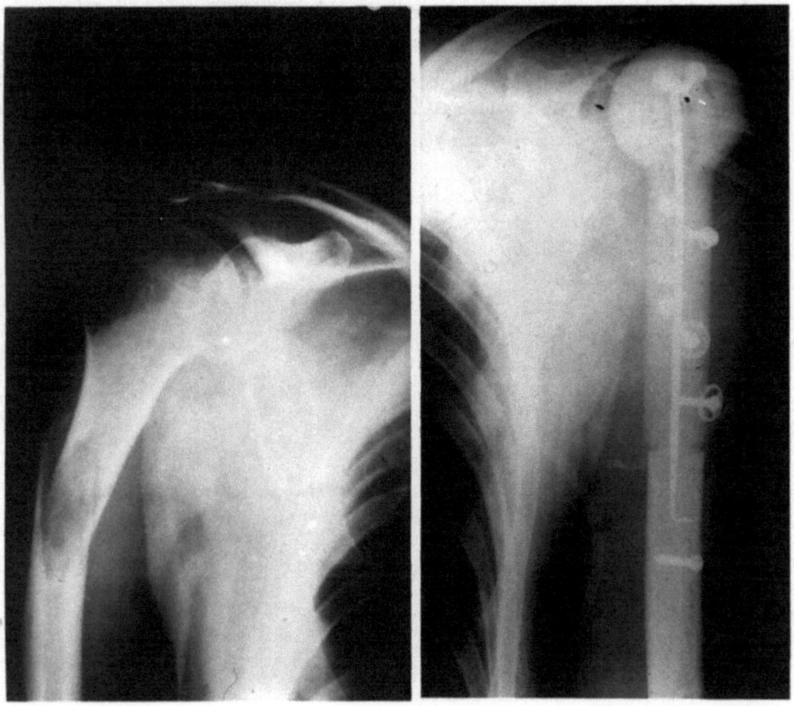

a b

Fig. 9a, b. Pathological proximal humerus fracture. Stabilization with an isoelastic prosthesis

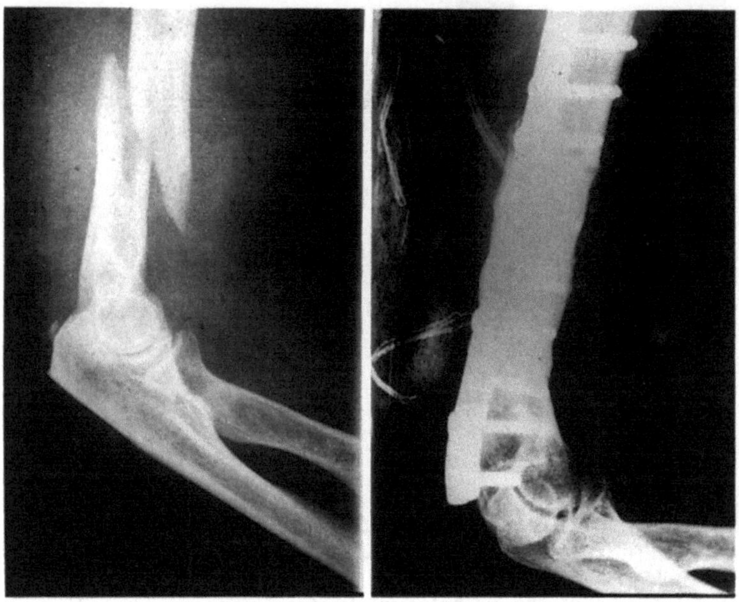

Fig. 10. Humerus shaft metastasis. Resection and simple plate compound osteosynthesis

internal fixator stabilization should be performed only in patients with a very short life expectancy [1].

The morbidity and mortality of these operations are low and the functional recovery very good. In our own series of 28 patients with spine metastases who

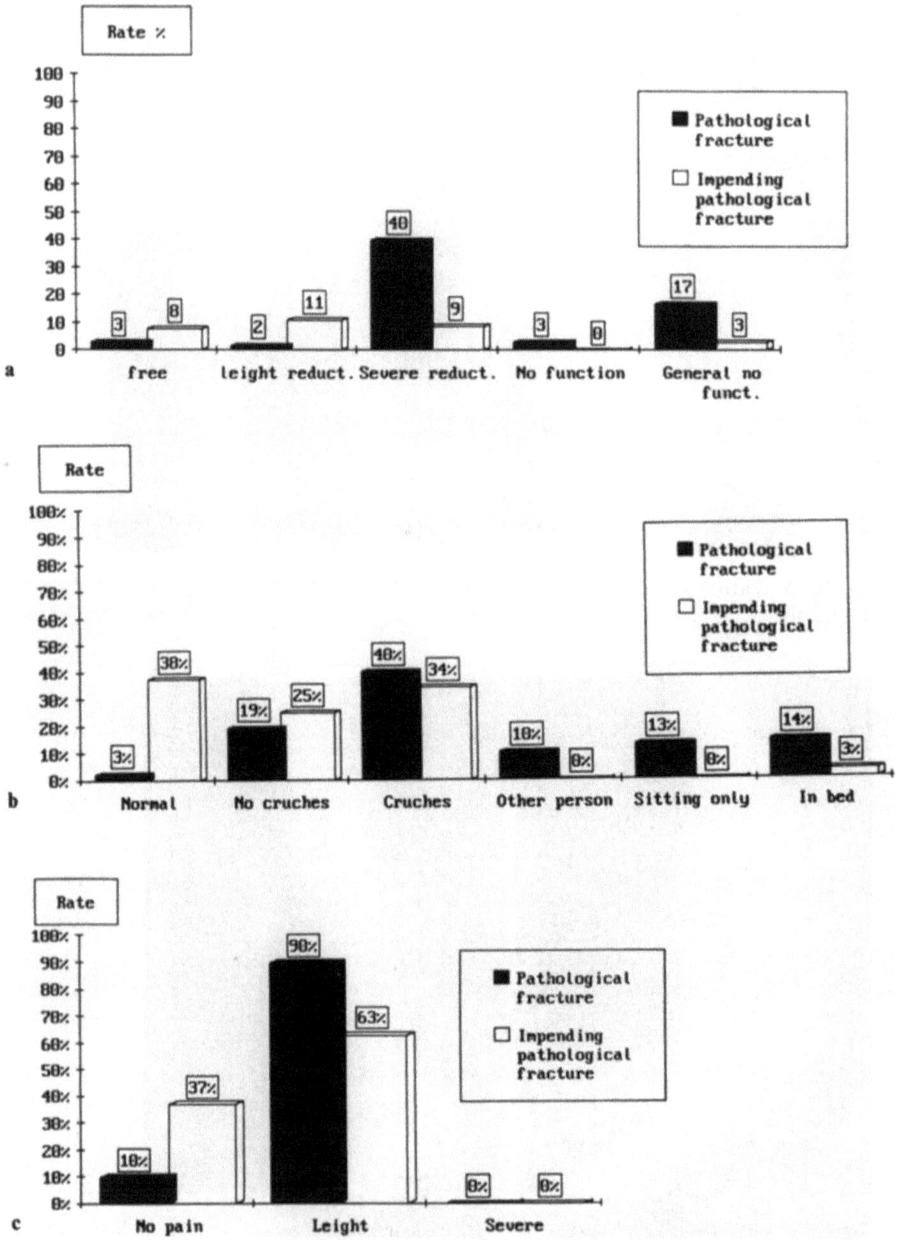

Fig. 11. Functional results of the pathological fracture management. **a** Function. **b** Mobilisation. **c** Pain

underwent surgical management between January 1990 and March 1992 there was no operation-related mortality. The 30-day mortality was 8%. No postoperative local complication and only one late implant dislocation was observed. Only one patient could not be mobilized postoperatively. No neurological complications were seen in these patients.

Pelvis metastases are common but pathological fractures rare. If the acetabulum or the load-bearing parts are affected, and radiotherapy is not effective, surgery must be considered, especially in younger patients with good general condition. Compound osteosynthesis techniques and acetabulum reconstruction plates are generally used. Internal hemipelvectomy and individual pelvis prosthesis reconstruction are rarely indicated in secondary tumors of the pelvis but should be considered in special cases.

In arm metastases the therapy regimen differs from that in the leg or trunk skeleton because here only function and not normal weight bearing must be restored. If the metastasis affects the proximal humerus, resection and isoelastic prosthesis replacement is used (Fig. 9). In shaft metastases resection and a compound single plate or compound locking nail osteosyntheses are performed (Fig. 10). Only in patients with a very short life expectancy can a locking nail without metastasis resection be performed. As in the femur, multiple unlocked nails should no longer be used because of insufficient stabilization and dislocation of the nail, especially after tumor progression.

Using this therapy regimen good or partial functional recovery can be obtained in nearly all patients. The results regarding function, mobilization, and pain are superior in patients with impending as opposed to actual pathological fractures (Fig. 11).

References

1. Everbeck V (1992) Die chirurgische Therapie von Knochenmetastasen der Wirbelsäule und des Beckens. Verhandlungsband des Symposiums: die chirurgische Therapie von Skelettmetastasen. Springer, Berlin Heidelberg New York
2. Friedl W, Ruf W, Krebs H (1986) Funktionelle Ergebnisse nach konservativer und operativer Therapie pathologischer Frakturen bei malignen Erkrankungen. Langenbecks Arch Chir 368: 185–196
3. Friedl W, Ruf W, Mischkowsky T (1986) Die Doppelplattenverbundosteosynthese bei subtrochanteren pathologischen Frakturen. Eine klinische und experimentelle Untersuchung. Chirurg 57: 713–718
4. Friedl W (1990) Indication, management and results of surgical therapy of pathological fractures in patients with bone metastases. Eur J Surg Oncol 16: 380–396
5. Friedl W (1992) Die Doppelplattenverbundosteosynthese. Ein Verfahren zur belastungsstabilen Versorgung des subtrochanteren bis supracondylären Femurbereiches. Aktuel Traumatol (in press)
6. Menck H, Schulze S, Larsen E (1988) Metastasis size in pathological fractures. Acta Orthop Scand 59: 151–154
7. Pizzaro G, Piva L, Mapelli S, Zucchi V (1991) Surgical treatment of distant metastases in renal cell carcinoma. Arch Ital Urol Nephrol Androl 63: 254–258
8. Pouilleart P, Beuzeboc P (1991) Value of clodronat in the treatment of bone metastases. Bull Cancer Paris 78: 737–741

Survival After Lung Surgery for Metastatic Renal Cancer

D. Branscheid[1], S. Pomer[2], S. Krysa[1], and I. Vogt-Moykopf[1]

Introduction

The lungs are the most frequent metastatic site (75% of all cases) [3, 9] and are typical of renal cancer dissemination along the vena cava. Biologically it makes sense to render the lung free of the tumor to prevent its further spread. Local excision of metastases is an effective form of treatment in patients with underlying renal cell carcinoma if only one distant organ is affected; solitary lung metastases occur in 1%–4% of all cases [14].

Khoury and Saul [7] have reviewed the data on survival after local excision of lung metastases. According to their data, survival after the removal of solitary metastases varied according to whether the lesion was concomitant (mean survival 18 months) or secondary to radical nephrectomy (mean survival 3 years).

Solitary metastasis is the best indication for surgery, although multiple lesions can also be excised [20]. Recently, promising results have been obtained with resection of bilateral metastases [5, 20]. The requirements for excision of lung metastases are otherwise (a) the ability to control the primary renal cancer, (b) the presence of metastases in one organ only, (c) local operability, and (d) a low risk of the surgical procedure. However, surgery is still controversial in cases with multiple organ involvement because of poor survival [2, 4]. With the advent of effective adjuvant treatment regimens, the indication for metastasectomy will hopefully soon become less restricted.

The preoperative evaluation of a patient with pulmonary metastatic renal cell carcinoma cannot be overemphasized. Computed tomography (CT), lung tomography, bronochoscopy, or mediastinoscopy may be needed for the proper assessment of metastases. The shortcomings of lung CT and lung tomography are apparent when the size and number of lesions are evaluated; in particular, the extent of metastases may be overestimated. Due to the low resolution of CT and lung tomography structures such as intrapulmonary lymph nodes, inflammations, and scars may be visualized and mistaken for metastatic lesions. Sternotomy has proven to offer the most suitable access to multiple bilateral lesions

[1] Thorax-Klinik, Amalienstr. 5, D-69126 Heidelberg, Germany
[2] Chirurgische Universitätsklinik, Abteilung Urologie, Im Neuenheimer Feld 110, D-69120 Heidelberg, Germany

and in cases with uncertain preoperative evidence of tumor origin and spread. Median sternotomy can easily be extended to median laparotomy for exploration of the abdominal cavity and retroperitoneum. Thus the obstacles encountered with lateral thoracotomy can be avoided. Transversal thoracotomy also has the advantage of possible bilateral exploration, and resection and is widely employed for this purpose.

Material and Methods

The study included 66 patients with metastatic renal cell carcinoma who had undergone surgery for their pulmonary lesions between 1 January 1972 and 31 December 1989. There were 46 men (70%) and 20 women (30%). The median age was 55 years (range 26–71): 48 patients (73%) were aged over 50 years and 18 (27%) under 50 years. Median sternotomy was used as operative access in 36 cases (55%).

A retrospective analysis was performed to examine factors with potential impact on survival. Survival was measured from the date of pulmonary operation to the date of death. Patients with mortality within 30 days after the operative were also included in the analysis. Survival curves were plotted and medians calculated using the Kaplan-Meier method [6]. Attention was focused on several potential prognostic variables. Univariate tests of significance were performed using the log rank test [6].

Results

Immediate Intra- and Postoperative Results

Lung metastases developed in 15 patients (24%) within 1 year after nephrectomy and in another 15 within 2.5 years. The time from diagnosis to development of metastases was over 2.5 years in 36 patients (52%) and in one patient was even 26 years. Solitary pulmonary metastases were found in 24 patients (36%), two to five metastases in 17 (26%), and six or more in 25 patients (38%). In the initial thoracic operations metastases were localized unilaterally in 42 (64%) and bilaterally in 24 (36%). Intraoperative evidence proved the preoperative estimate of number of lesions correct in 49% of cases; in 28% more lesions and in 23% fewer lesions estimated preoperatively were found at surgery.

Radical metastasectomy was performed in 55 (77%) thoracotomies. In 16 patients (23%) complete resection of metastases could not be achieved, mainly as a result of severe mediastinal and/or bronchial involvement. Anatomic and atypical segment or subsegment resections were performed in 65% of operations. Only one enucleation was carried out. Lobectomies and bilobectomies were performed in 31% of cases. In only 3% of cases did the metastasectomy lead to pneumonectomy. Mediastinal lymph nodes were involved in 15% of patients with lung metastases. The 30-day mortality was 4.5% ($n = 3$); the causes were empyema, bleeding, and respiratory failure.

Follow-Up Results

The cumulative 5-year survival rate was 37% – superior to the 30% in all 549 patients treated by surgery for pulmonary metastatic disease of other origin. The 1-year and 3-year survival rates in the group of patients with renal cancer were 74% and 47%, respectively. Figure 1 presents the overall survival curve, and Table 1 shows the survival rates in terms of the clinical characteristics that were examined. Patients after radical metastasectomy had a better prognosis (median survival 823 days, 5-year survival 41%) than after a resection classified as noncurative. No influence of sex on prognosis was found. Age did prove to be of importance, as older patients (over 50 years) had a better prognosis than younger ones ($p = 0.137$); their median survival was 1482 days and 5-year survival rate 50% (Fig. 2). The time from initial diagnosis to development of metastasis was predictive for survival; patients who had evidence of metastasis within 2.5 years after nephrectomy had a poorer prognosis than those who developed metastatic lesions later (Fig. 3). Neither the number of metastatic sites (Fig. 4) nor uni- or bilateral involvement (Fig. 5) were important prognostic factors. Lung parenchyma sparing resections yielded the best results. The involvement of intrathoracic and mediastinal lymph nodes did not lead to significantly poorer prognosis; however, it confirmed the negative trend in terms of poorer survival of

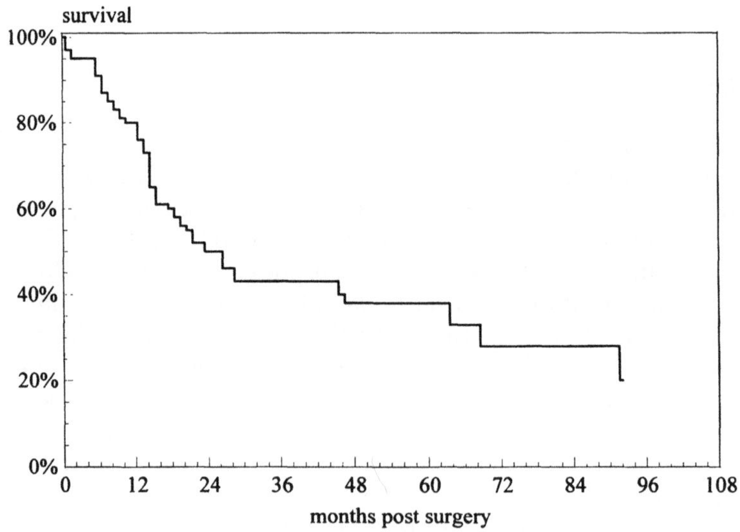

Fig. 1. Overall survival rate after surgery for renal cell carcinoma with pulmonary metastases

Table 1. Survival rates after lung surgery for metastatic renal cell carcinoma

	1-year (%)	3-year (%)	5-year (%)	Median (days)
Time from initial diagnosis to development of metastasis				
Under 2.5 years	71	30	0	672
Over 2.5 years	79	67	58	2112
Number of pulmonary metastatic lesions				
One	71	57	38	1446
Two to five	71	41	ND	795
Six or more	80	40	ND	823
Uni-/bilateral involvement				
Unilateral	76	48	40	439
Bilateral	75	44	ND	823
Lymph node involvement				
Without	75	48	42	823
With	72	47	23	672
Adjuvant chemo-/radiotherapy of metastatic lesion				
Without	74	50	36	1446
With	75	38	ND	667
Adjuvant chemo-/radiotherapy of primary tumor				
Without	81	53	45	1446
With	58	33	23	439

ND, No data.

these patients (Fig. 6). Prior systemic chemotherapy or local radiotherapy of the metastatic lesion (Fig. 7) or the primary tumor (Fig. 8) was associated with poorer 5-year survival (23% versus 45%), possibly demonstrating the influence of the advanced stage of the underlying renal cancer.

Discussion

Basic Benefits of Surgical Approach

The basic value of surgery for lung metastasis as opposed to other approaches can best be appreciated by keeping in mind the natural history of the affected patients. Generally the 5-year survival rate in metastatic renal cancer is 0%–15% [2, 3, 9–12]. However, in our patients the rate was 37% and reached even 41% in the group with metastases classified as radically resected. Median survival after diagnosis of metastases averaged 8 months in this study.

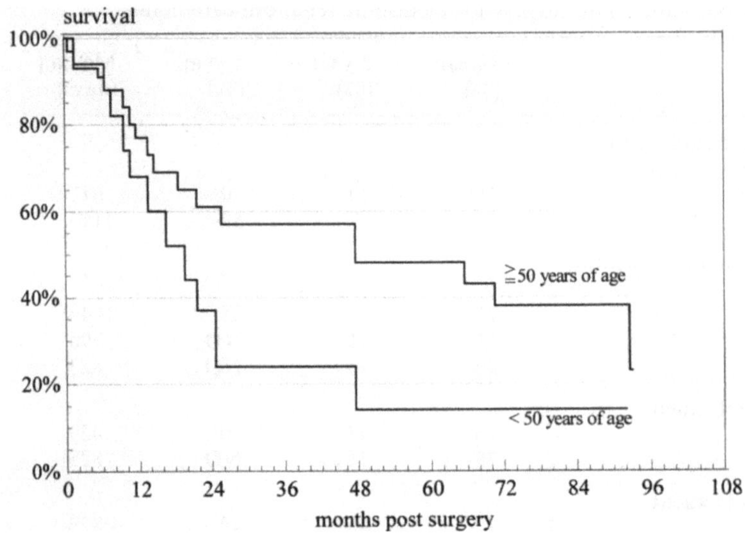

Fig. 2. Age and survival rate after lung surgery for metastatic renal cell carcinoma

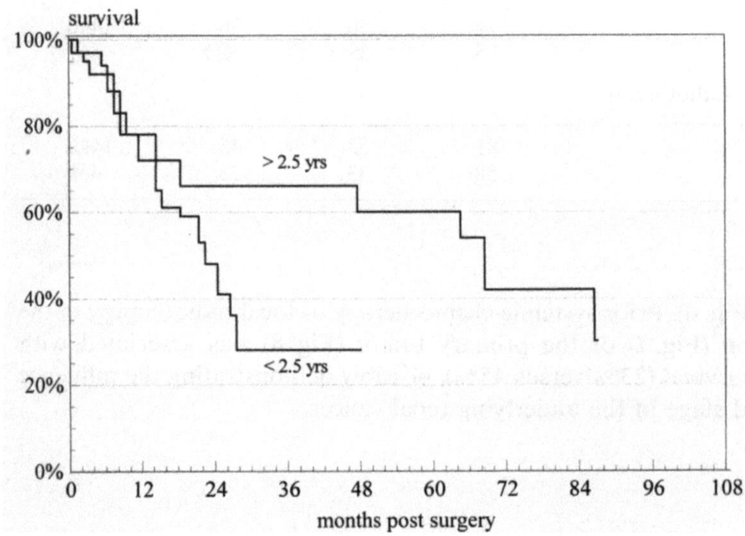

Fig. 3. Time from initial diagnosis to the development of metastases and survival rate after lung surgery for metastatic renal cell carcinoma

Selection of Patients for Surgical Treatment of Lung Metastases

This study investigated renal cell carcinoma patients with pulmonary metastases treated by surgery to identify clinical characteristics prognostic for survival. The results may offer an aid in the selection of patients for surgical

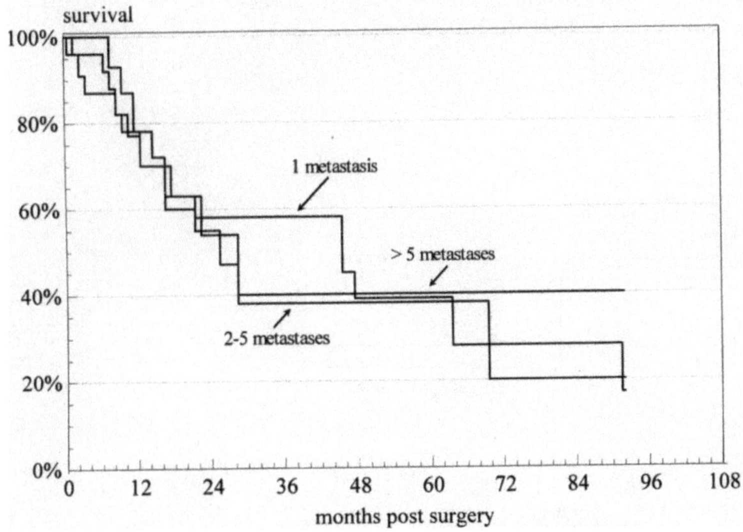

Fig. 4. Number of pulmonary metastatic lesions and survival rate after lung surgery for metastatic renal cell carcinoma

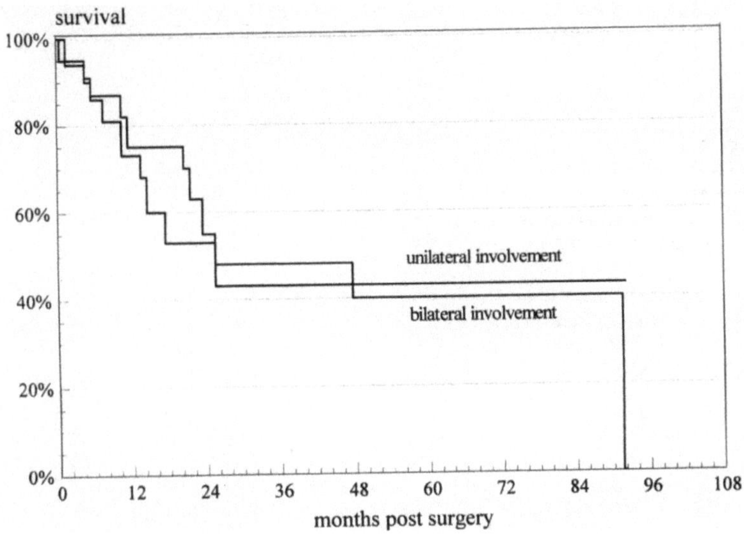

Fig. 5. Unilateral/bilateral involvement and survival rate after lung surgery for metastatic renal cell carcinoma

treatment. The number of lesions and unilateral/bilateral involvement proved to be of no prognostic significance. The positive course of patients with a long disease-free interval between the time of nephrectomy and diagnosis of pulmonary metastases (> 2.5 years) is not negatively affected after metastasectomy [4]. Their survival, 58% in this study, was comparable to that found in patients

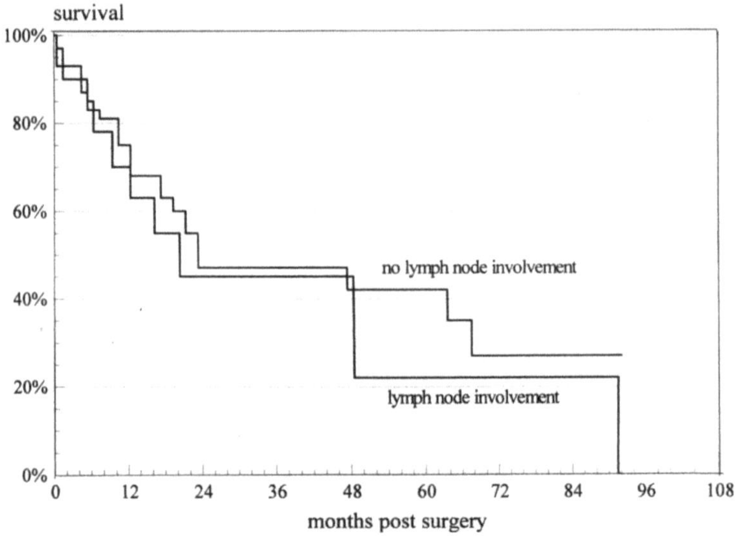

Fig. 6. Lymph node involvement and survival rate after lung surgery for metastatic renal cell carcinoma

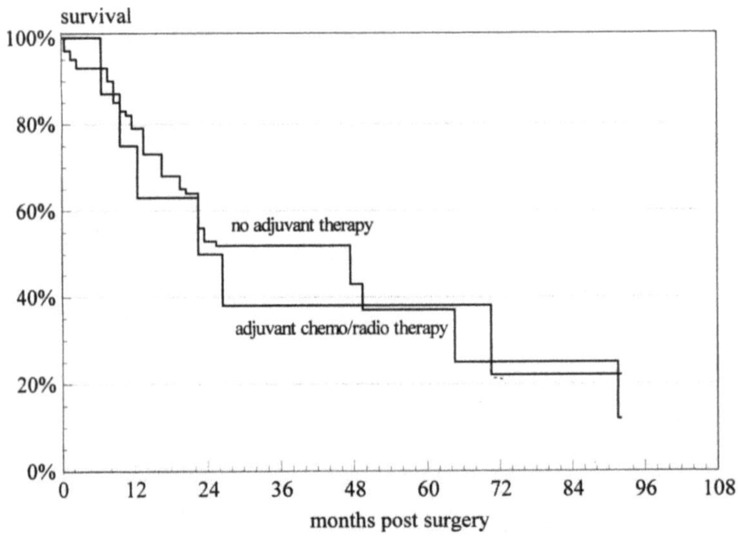

Fig. 7. Adjuvant chemo-/radiotherapy of the metastatic lesion and survival rate after lung surgery for metastatic renal cell carcinoma

without metastases [3]. A poorer prognosis was found in patients with simultaneous diagnosis of renal cancer and pulmonary metastases or metastastic development in a shorter (<2 years) postnephrectomy period. Long-term postmetastasectomy remissions were more frequent in patients over 50 years of age.

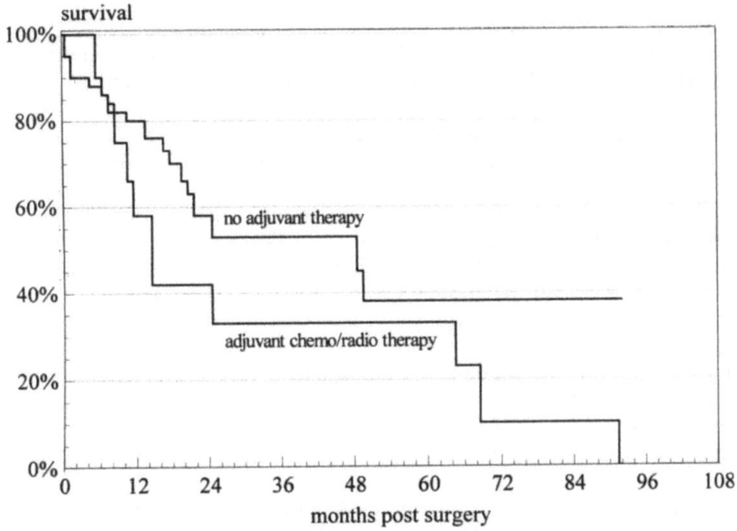

Fig. 8. Adjuvant chemo-/radiotherapy of the primary tumor and survival rate after lung surgery for metastatic renal cell carcinoma

Value of Lung Surgery in the Interdisciplinary Concept for Treatment of Renal Cell Carcinoma Metastases

With the advent of recombinant interferon-α [13] and since promising results have been obtained with immunotherapy using this and interleukin-2 [18], the role of surgery for lung metastases has changed and is awaiting a possible reassessment. Obviously immunotherapy can have a substantial impact on the course of the metastatic disease, with remission rates around 20%–25% for cytokine combination regimens [1, 17, 19]. Some publications focus on the outcome of immunotherapy in cases classified as stable disease over prolonged periods of time [15]. Clinical experience suggests that such long periods of stable disease characterized by a tolerable general condition show neither dramatic, measurable response nor signs of progression. There is also some evidence of survival advantage in these patients [15]. Patients showing partial responses, with more than 50% regression of lung metastases, are candidates for surgical removal of residual tumors. Surprisingly, these so-called surgical complete remissions have proven to be long lasting. In a recent meta-analysis on 30 such patients, 90% remained free of tumor for several years after metastasectomy [8].

References

1. Atzpodien J, Körfer A, Franks CR, Pollwod AH, Kirchner H (1990) Home therapy with rIL2 and IFN-alpha-2b in advanced human malignancies. Lancet 335: 1509–1512
2. De Forges A, Rey A, Klink M, Ghosn M, Kramar A, Droz JP (1988) Prognostic factors of adult metastatic renal carcinoma: a multivariate analysis. Semin Surg Oncol 4: 149–154
3. De Kernion JB, Ramming KP, Smith RB (1978) The natural history of metastatic renal cell carcinoma: a computer analysis. J Urol 120: 148–152
4. Elson PJ, Witte RS, Trump DL (1988) Prognostic factors for survival in patients with recurrent or metastatic renal cell carcinoma. Cancer Res 48: 7310–7313
5. Jett JR, Hollinger CG, Zinsmeister AR, Pairolero PC (1983) Pulmonary resection of metastatic renal cell carcinoma. Chest 84: 442
6. Kaplan EL, Meier P (1958) Non-parametric estimation from incomplete observation. J Am Statistical Assoc 53: 457–481
7. Khoury S, Saul A (1986) Metastatic renal adenocarcinoma. In: De Kernion JB, Pavone-Macaluso M (eds) Tumors of the kidney. Williams and Wilkins, Baltimore, pp 194–294
8. Kim B, Louie AC (1992) Surgical resection following interleukin-2-therapy for metastatic renal cell carcinoma prolongs remission. Arch Surg 127: 1343–1349
9. Maldazys JG, De Kernion JB (1986) Prognostic factors in metastatic renal carcinoma. J Urol 136: 376–379
10. Mc Nichols DW, Segura JW, De Weerd JH (1981) Renal cell carcinoma. Long-term survival and late recurrence. J Urol 126: 17–23
11. Middleton RG (1967) Surgery for metastatic renal cell carcinoma. J Urol 97: 973–979
12. Montie JE, Stewart BH, Straffon RA, Banowsky LHW, Hewitt CB, Montague DK (1977) The role of adjunctive nephrectomy in patients with metastatic renal cell carcinoma. J Urol 117: 376–379
13. Muss HB (1987) Interferon therapy for renal cell carcinoma. Semin Oncol 14: 36–42
14. O'Dea MJ, Zincke H, Utz DC, Bernatz BE (1978) The treatment of renal cell carcinoma with solitary metastasis. J Urol 120: 540–542
15. Palmer PA, Vinke J, Philip T, Negrier S, Atzpodien J, Kirchner H, Oskam R, Franks CR (1992) Prognostic factors for survival in patients with advanced renal cell carcinoma treated with recombinant interleukin-2. Ann Oncol 3: 475–480
16. Peto R, Peto J (1972) Asymptomatically efficient rank invariant test procedures. J R Statistical Soc A 135: 185–206
17. Pomer S, Thiele R, Daniel V, Weimer R, Löhrke H, Schirrmacher V, Staehler G (1991) Sequential treatment of patients with advanced renal cell carcinoma with autologous tumor vaccine and subcutanous administration of recombinant interleukin 2 and interferon alpha-2b. World J Urol 9: 223–227
18. Rosenberg SA, Lotze MT, Mule JJ (1988) New approaches to the immunotherapy of cancer using interleukin-2. Ann Intern Med 108: 853–864
19. Rosenberg SA, Lotze MT, Yang JC (1989) Combination therapy with IL-2 and IFN-alpha for the treatment of patients with advanced cancer. J Clin Oncol 7: 1726–1732
20. Vogt-Moykopf I, Meyer G (1986) Surgical technique in operations for pulmonary metastases. J Thorac Cardiovasc Surg 34: 125–132
21. West WH, Tauer KN, Yannelli JR (1987) Constant-infusion rIL2 in adoptive immunotherapy of advanced cancer. N Engl J Med 316: 898–905

Partial Nephrectomy for Renal Cell Carcinoma: Clinical and Biological Considerations

E.A. Klein

Partial nephrectomy for the treatment of renal tumors dates to the late 1800s. Recent enthusiasm for renal-sparing surgery has been stimulated by the development of renal angiography, experience with renal vascular surgery for treatment of renal artery stenosis and other diseases, improved methods for preventing renal ischemic damage, the growing incidence of incidentally discovered low-stage renal tumors [1], and good long-term survival in early series of patients treated by partial nephrectomy [2]. Continued experience has established that partial nephrectomy can be performed safely with low morbidity and good preservation of renal function and can provide long-term cures of renal cancer. While radical nephrectomy is the procedure of choice for the curative excision of localized renal cell carcinoma, partial nephrectomy is indicated in patients in whom radical nephrectomy would result in the need for renal replacement therapy in the form of renal dialysis or transplantation.

Patient Selection

Partial nephrectomy for the treatment of renal cell carcinoma should be considered in any of six situations: (a) bilateral synchronous renal tumors, (b) cancer in an anatomically or functionally solitary kidney, (c) unilateral tumors in patients with a functioning contralateral kidney and a concomitant condition with the potential for adversely affecting future renal function, (d) unilateral tumors in patients with a functioning but impaired contralateral kidney, (e) renal cell carcinoma in von Hippel-Lindau disease (VHL), and (f) treatment of small tumors discovered incidentally by abdominal imaging studies.

Bilateral synchronous renal cell carcinoma is the most frequent indication for partial nephrectomy [3]. The philosophy in approaching these tumors has been to attempt to preserve as much functioning renal tissue as possible. Generally this means performing bilateral partial nephrectomies whenever possible, usually as staged procedures. When a large tumor on one side precludes partial nephrectomy, a radical nephrectomy is performed on the more

Section of Urologic Oncology, Cleveland Clinic Foundation, 9500 Euclid Avenue, Cleveland, OH 44195, USA involved side with a contralateral partial nephrectomy. In the case of bilateral partial nephrectomies that on the easier side is performed first; if radical nephrectomy is indicated on one side, the partial nephrectomy is performed first. This approach obviates the need for temporary dialysis in the immediate postoperative period if ischemic renal dysfunction occurs on the operated side. This is also the most flexible approach for planning the procedure on the opposite side; occasionally a partial rather than a radical nephrectomy is performed on the second side when the initial procedure results in a remnant kidney of insufficient size to avoid dialysis.

Unilateral renal tumors in functionally or anatomically solitary kidneys are the second most frequent indication for partial nephrectomy [3]. In these cases a functioning contralateral kidney is lacking, increasing the potential need for acute dialysis in the postoperative period owing to ischemic-induced acute tubular necrosis of the operated kidney. A renal remnant of at least 25% of a normal kidney is necessary to avoid permanent renal failure.

Unilateral renal tumors with functionally impaired contralateral kidneys also occur with some frequency. Contralateral functional impairment can result from a variety of conditions including renal artery disease, hydronephrosis, chronic pyelonephritis, and nephrosclerosis. The operative considerations in these patients are similar to those with anatomically solitary kidneys.

Another indication for partial nephrectomy is in patients with unilateral tumors and a normally functioning opposite kidney which is affected by a condition which potentially threatens its function. This may include renal calculi, renal artery stenosis, azotemia, diabetes mellitus, or hypertension. The presence of such conditions is a relative indication for partial nephrectomy, although the decision to perform a partial nephrectomy must be individualized by considering the extent of tumor, difficulty of partial resection, life expectancy, and ultimate threat to renal function if unilateral total nephrectomy is performed. The relative merits of partial nephrectomy in patients with contralateral stone disease has diminished with the advent of nonsurgical and metabolic approaches to the treatment of stones.

The rationale for partial nephrectomy in patients with VHL is based upon a younger average age of presentation versus typical renal cell carcinoma (resulting in longer potential life span) and the propensity for the renal tumors of VHL to be both multifocal and bilateral [4, 5]. However, because of the genetic nature of VHL, patients treated by partial nephrectomy are at high risk for new tumors as well as the usual risk for local recurrences due to inadequate excision [5]. These patients must be followed carefully and advised of the potential need for repeat renal surgery which may result in total loss of renal function. Previous studies have suggested a 30%–35% risk of tumor progression and death from renal cancer in VHL [6]. The risk of progression or death following partial nephrectomy in these patients is undefined.

The role of partial nephrectomy in patients with unilateral tumors and normal contralateral kidneys is controversial [7]. This question is increasingly important with the widespread use of abdominal computed tomographic (CT) and ultrasound resulting in the growing discovery of unsuspected renal tumors

[1]. Most of these incidentally discovered tumors are asymptomatic, small, found on the peripheral surface of the kidney, and of low pathological stage. Surgical excision of tumors of such small volume should in most cases effect cure. However, whether this is best accomplished by partial or by total nephrectomy is not defined. Several factors argue in favor of radical nephrectomy in this situation: (a) the low ultimate risk of contralateral renal loss as defined in long term follow-up studies of living related donor nephrectomy patients [8], (b) the low risk (1%–2%) of developing a metachronous contralateral renal tumor, (c) a 10% local recurrence rate after partial nephrectomy as compared to 1%–2% for radical nephrectomy [3], and (d) occasional cases of unsuspected mutifocal tumors which would not be removed by partial nephrectomy [9].

In favor of partial nephrectomy is recent evidence of the risk of hyperfiltration injury in patients with solitary kidneys and the ease with which partial nephrectomy can be performed with good margins for small, peripherally located tumors. Several animal studies have demonstrated that loss of functioning renal tissue results in hypertrophy and hyperfiltration of the remaining nephrons [10, 11]. These adaptive phenomena lead to increases in glomerular capillary flow and hydrostatic pressure and in cases of substantial renal loss can lead to glomerular sclerosis and renal failure [12, 13]. Novick et al. have recently reported that patients with less than one kidney remaining after surgery are at increased risk for the development of proteinuria, glomerulopathy, and renal failure [14].

In the case of an incidentally discovered peripheral renal tumor partial nephrectomy can usually be performed without loss of more than 10%–15% of renal mass. The resulting increase in glomuler filtration rate (GFR) per nephron is theoretically less after partial than radical nephrectomy because total GFR is distributed over more functioning nephrons (85% versus 50%) and should yield more protection against hyperfiltration-induced injury. Ultimately the choice of treatment of small tumors with a normal contralateral kidney depends on long-term studies which define both the chance of cure with partial nephrectomy versus the risk of hyperfiltration-induced renal failure after radical nephrectomy. Presently available data suggest that both the risk of local recurrence after partial nephrectomy and the risk of renal failure after unilateral nephrectomy are small, so that treatment choices still should be individualized based on operative considerations and patient choice. Whether dietary interventions such as protein restriction will further reduce the risk of hyperfiltration-induced injury after nephrectomy, and how this will impact on treatment choice must await the results of longitudinal studies.

Preoperative Evaluation

A successful partial nephrectomy with negative surgical margins and presentation of kidney function is predicated on obtaining a good three-dimensional image of the involved kidney preoperatively. This necessitates visualizing the location of the tumor within the kidney and its relationship to both the renal vasculature and the collecting system. Tumor location, size, and depth of penetration toward the hilum are best demonstrated by CT. Magnetic resonance imaging (MRI) is not as sensitive in defining intrarenal anatomy or the presence of lymph node enlargement as CT and is not routinely employed.

The relationship of the tumor to the renal vasculature is best determined by renal angiography. This reveals the number and location of the main renal arteries and the location of the arterial branches supplying both the tumor and uninvolved kidney. Digital subtraction angiography usually does not visualize renal artery branches in sufficient detail to be useful for partial nephrectomy. Increasingly sophisticated MRI techniques may one day replace the need for renal angiography in defining the main renal artery and its first-order branches. Renal venography or MRI may be used preoperatively to define the extent of thrombus within the renal vein if not clearly determined by angiography.

The relationship of the tumor to the collecting system and the part of the kidney to be preserved is best determined by intravenous urogram or retrograde pyelogram.

Operative Considerations

A variety of surgical techniques for partial nephrectomy have been described, including enucleation, polar segmental nephrectomy after ligation of the corresponding renal arterial branch, wedge resection, major transverse resection, and extracorporeal partial nephrectomy with autotransplantation. The detailed technical aspects of each of these procedures have been previously described [15].

The basic surgical principles for partial nephrectomy are (a) early vascular control, (b) preservation of function of the operated kidney without ischemic damage, (c) complete tumor excision with negative surgical margins, (d) watertight closure of the collecting system, (e) careful hemostasis, and (f) closure of the renal defect with perirenal fat or hemostatic sponge.

All but the largest centrally located tumors can be removed by in situ partial nephrectomy without the need for bench repair and autotransplantation. An extraperitoneal flank incision through the bed of the 11th or 12th rib is used routinely for in situ cases. This incision allows easy access to all parts of the kidney and renal vasculature while allowing the operation to be done at skin level. The kidney is first mobilized outside of Gerota's fascia, and perirenal fat is then cleared down to the surface of the kidney. The fat overlying the tumor is left undisturbed.

Some small peripheral tumors can be excised without the need for occlusion of the renal artery, although regional hypothermia with renal artery occlusion is generally used for all cases. This permits approximately 3 h of operative time while protecting the kidney from ischemic damage. The mobilized kidney is placed within a plastic bowel bag which is gathered around the renal sinus. Lap sponges are placed outside of the bag to protect adjacent organs from ice slush. Prior to renal artery occlusion 12.5 g mannitol is infused via a peripheral intravenous line for additional protection against renal ischemia. The renal artery is occluded with an atraumatic vascular clamp, and the kidney is immediately covered with sterile ice slush. The kidney is left packed in ice for 15 min to allow a core temperature of 15°–20°C to be reached before tumor excision is begun. The main renal vein is left unoccluded to allow some degree of renal oxygenation and identification of "back bleeders" on the cut surface of the kidney.

The choice of technique for tumor excision depends on its size, location, and relationship to the renal vessels and collecting system. For most tumors on the surface of the kidney or those which do not extend deeply into the hilum wedge excision is the procedure of choice. This is the simplest procedure and avoids the need for an extensive hilar dissection. A 1- to 2-cm margin of normal kidney is excised along with the tumor. Frozen section examination of the margin of the specimen should be obtained to ensure complete tumor excision. Following excision the collecting system is closed with absorbable suture, and bleeders are oversewn with 4–0 chromic. The argon beam coagulator may serve as a useful adjunct to help control small bleeders on the cut surface of the renal cortex. The renal parenchyma is then reapproximated over oxycel using interrupted 2–0 chromic sutures. The clamp on the renal artery is then removed and the kidney surface irrigated with warm saline. The raw cortical surface is observed for a few minutes to ensure adequate hemostasis, and the kidney is then covered with perirenal fact. A penrose drain is placed through a separate stab incision through the flank.

Because of the risk of incomplete tumor excision with microscopically positive surgical margins documented by several reports [16, 17], simple enucleation for small lesions on the surface of the kidney is reserved for the multiple cystic tumors seen in VHL [5].

Segmental polar nephrectomy and major transverse resections are variations of the same technique. The general principles are similar to those outlined for wedge resection, but branches of the renal artery may be dissected and ligated prior to tumor excision. This helps to define the margin of excision and further reduces blood loss.

Lesions with renal venous invasion by tumor thrombus present a special surgical challenge. The presence of renal vein thrombus is often associated with more aggressive tumors. In a series of nine patients with renal vein thrombi undergoing partial nephrectomy two had perinephric fat invasion, and four died of metastatic renal cancer, including two with concurrent local recurrences [18]. These tumors are more difficult to excise and may carry a higher risk of operative ischemia time as well as an increased likelihood of the need for ex vivo excision. This results in an increased incidence of acute tubular necrosis, with three of the patients in this series requiring temporary dialysis.

Large renal tumors located in the renal hilum also present a special challenge. Whenever possible these tumors are excised by an in situ approach, because the use of ex vivo bench excision with autotransplantation is associated with a higher chance of temporary and permanent renal failure [3]. When ex vivo excision is necessary, an extrafascial radical nephrectomy is performed initially. The artery and vein are transected as the last steps prior to removal of the kidney in order to minimize warm ischemia time, and the blood supply to the upper ureter must be carefully preserved. We prefer to transect the ureter and perform tumor excision on a separate sterile workbench. This permits precise excision of the tumor, facilitates any necessary vascular reconstruction, and allows simultaneous preparation of the iliac fossa for transplantation by a second surgical team. Following removal the kidney is immediately flushed with an ice-cold electrolyte solution and placed in a basin filled with sterile ice slush. This allows completion of all bench work while minimizing the risks of ischemic damage. Following tumor excision the artery and veins are flushed to look for unsuspected leaks. The remaining kidney is then transplanted into the iliac fossa using standard techniques. We routinely reestablish ureteral continuity by ureteroureterostomy over a stent.

Outcome and Survival after Partial Nephrectomy

After complete excision of tumor the goal of partial nephrectomy is the preservation of renal function without the need for dialysis or renal transplantation. In a series of 100 consecutive partial nephrectomies at our institution, 93 patients had immediate return of renal function postoperatively, 4 had delayed return of function requiring temporary dialysis, and only 3 suffered permanent nonfunction [3]. Serum creatinine levels in the patients with preserved renal functioned ranged from 0.9 to 4.6 mg/dl, with a mean of 1.76 mg/dl. The use of ex vivo excision with autotransplantation was associated with a higher risk of both initial (36%) and permanent nonfunction (14%). Similarly, the presence of a renal vein thrombus also increased the need for temporary dialysis (33%) [18]. As already discussed, patients with less than one kidney remaining after surgery are at higher risk for the development of proteinuria, progressive glomerulopathy, and end-stage renal disease. There is a clear relationship in these patients between the risk of developing these problems and the amount of residual kidney and the length of time since surgery [14].

The development of renal failure in any patient after partial nephrectomy may have a significant impact on life-style and well mortality. The 1-, 2-, and 5-year survival rates for patients aged 55–64 years while on dialysis following radical nephrectomy for renal cell carcinoma in solitary kidney are 84%, 67%, and 33%, respectively, and fall to 73%, 51%, and 16% in patients older than 64 years [19]. These patients would have to survive disease-free on dialysis for 12–24 months prior to any consideration of renal transplantation. Furthermore, even a mild impairment of renal function would prevent patients who develop metastatic disease from being treated with currently available chemotherapy or immunotherapy regimens.

Survival after partial nephrectomy is influenced by tumor stage, the occurrence of bilateral tumors, the presence of local recurrences, and the presence of venous invasion [3]. In the series of patients from our institution, the overall 5-year survival was 67% and disease specific survival 84% [3]. Pathological stage I tumors had an overall 5-year survival of 73% and a cancer-specific survival of 90% (Table 1); the cancer-specific survival was statistically significantly better than that in stage III and IV tumors. Similarly, unilateral tumors had an overall 5-year survival of 77% and a cancer-specific survival of 97% (Table 2). This was statistically significantly better than bilateral tumors which presented synchronously or asynchronously (Table 2) and held true even when higher stage tumors were excluded (Table 1), suggesting that bilateral tumors are biologically more aggressive.

Local recurrences also impact adversely on survival. Of nine patients with local recurrences after partial nephrectomy, only two (22%) were alive and disease free at the time of last follow-up [3]. This observation emphasizes the

Table 1. Partial nephrectomy: 5-year survival by stage

	n	Overall (%)	Cancer specific (%)
State I	75	73	90*
Unilateral	37	80	100*
Bilateral synchronous	22	71	79
Bilateral asynchronous	16	67	82
Stage II	9	–	–
Stage III	10	68	76
Stage IV	6	22	41
Total	100	67	84

* $p < 0.05$.

Table 2. Partial nephrectomy: 5-year survival independent of stage

	n	Overall (%)	Cancer specific (%)
Unilateral	44	77	97*
Bilateral synchronous	28	73	82
Bilateral asynchronous	28	5	68
Total	100	67	84

* $p < 0.05$.

need to excise a wide margin of normal tissue in order to obtain complete tumor excision and negative surgical margins at the time of surgery. Similarly the presence of venous invasion, which typically indicates a more advanced local stage, was associated with a 44% cancer-related mortality at 17–47 months after surgery [18].

References

1. Konnak JW, Grossman HB (1985) Renal cell carcinoma as an incidental finding. J Urol 134: 1094
2. Topley M, Novick AC, Montie JE (1984) Long-term results following partial nephrectomy for localized renal adenocarcinoma. J Urol 131: 1050
3. Novick AC, Streem S, Montie JE et al. (1989) Conservative surgery for renal cell carcinoma: a single-center experience with 100 patients. J Urol 141: 835
4. Spencer WF, Novick AC, Montie JE et al. (1988) Surgical treatment of localized renal cell carcinoma in von Hippel-Lindau's disease. J Urol 139: 507
5. Klein EA, Novick AC (1990) Urologic manifestations of von Hippel-Lindau disease. AUA Update Ser 9: 257
6. Horton WA, Wong V, Eldridge R et al. (1976) von Hippel-Lindau disease: clinical and pathological manifestations in nine families with 50 affected members. Arch Intern Med 136: 769
7. Klein EA, Novick AC (1992) Partial nephrectomy for renal cell carcinoma. In: Lytton B (ed) Advances in urology. 5: 1
8. Weiland D, Sutherland DER, Chavers B et al. (1984) Information of 628 living related kidney donors at a single institution, with long term follow up in 472 cases. Transplant Proc 16: 5
9. Mukamel E, Konichezky M, Englestein D, Servadio C (1988) Incidental small renal tumors accompanying clinically overt renal cell carcinoma. J Urol 140: 22
10. Hostetter TH, Olson JL, Rennke HG et al. (1981) Hyperfiltration in remnant nephrons: a potentially adverse response to renal ablation. Am J Physiol 241: F85–F93
11. Shimamura T, Morrison AB (1975) A progressive glomerulosclerosis occurring in partial five-sixth nephrectomized rats. Am J Pathol 9: 95
12. Brenner BM (1983) Hemodynamically mediated glomerular injury and the progressive nature of kidney disease. Kidney Int 23: 647
13. Sugino N, Duffy G, Gulyassy PF (1967) Renal function after unilateral nephrectomy in normal man. Clin Res 15: 143
14. Novick AC, Gephardt G, Guz B et al. (1991) Long-term follow-up after partial removal of a solitary kidney. N Engl J Med 325: 1058
15. Novick AC (1987) Partial nephrectomy for renal cell carcinoma. Urol Clin North Am 14: 419
16. Smith RB, deKernion JB, Ehrlich RM et al. (1984) Bilateral renal cell carcinima and renal cell carcinoma in the solitary kidney. J Urol 132: 450
17. Marshall F, Taxy JB, Fishman EK et al. (1986) The feasibility of surgical enucleation for renal cell carcinoma. J Urol 135: 231
18. Angermeier KW, Novick AC, Streem SB, Montie JE (1990) Nephron-sparing surgery for renal cell carcinoma with venous involvement. J Urol 144: 1352
19. National Institutes of Health (1989) US Renal Data System, 1989 annual data report. Bethesda, Maryland, August 1989

Investigation of the Tumor Capsule in Renal Cell Carcinoma and Its Significance for Treatment

W. de Riese[1], E.P. Allhoff[2], S. Liedke[2], C.G. Stief[2], M. Werner[3], H. Kirchner[4], J. Atzpodien[4], and E. Reale[5]

Introduction

Nearly all human renal cell carcinomas (RCC) are found to be encapsuled [3]. Histological assessment using conventional staining techniques such as hematoxylin and eosin (H&E) reveals a capsule surrounding the tumor which might act as a barrier between normal and malignant tissue. However, the exact origin and function of this capsule is unknown. In 1925 Lubarsch was the first to describe renal tumors exhibiting tumor capsules [7]. He called this tissue structure a pseudocapsule. Up to now investigations concerning this tissue phenomenon have been very rare.

In the course of a histomorphological study on the localization of proteoglycans in different human organs, tumor-bearing kidneys were fixed by vascular perfusion immediately after their complete or partial surgical removal for malignancy [5]. During the vascular perfusion of the specimens for electron microscopy it was observed that renal tumors were not perfused by the fixative solution. The tumors were sharply delineated from the surrounding normal parenchyma by a compact capsule which apparently prevented the progression of the fixative dye solution. The presence of this compact capsule surrounding malignant renal tumors is commonly described in the routine pathological histology, but even up to now the interpretation of its structure, nature, and tumor-related function is still controversial, as outlined by the authors in a recent report [9].

To clarify the function of this tumor-related histomorphological structure we analyzed specimens of previously untreated RCC patients by comparing immunohistochemical and electron microscopic findings.

[1] Marienhospital II, Urologische Klinik der Universität Bochum, Widumer Str. 6, D-44627 Herne, Germany, Medizinische Hochschule, [2] Klinik für Urologie, [3] Abteilung Zytogenetik und Immunhistochemie, Pathologisches Institut, [4] Abteilung Medizinische Onkologie, [5] Abteilung Zellbiologie und Elektronenmikroskop, Zentrum Anatomie; Konstanty-Gutschow-Str. 8, D-30625 Hannover, Germany

Material and Methods

Thirteen consecutive cases of renal cell carcinomas were analyzed. Table 1 presents the histomorphological characteristics of the investigated tumors. Not only in early (e.g., patient 11) but also in advanced stages (e.g., patient 13) a tumor capsule was found. Immediately after conventional radical nephrectomy the tumor-bearing kidneys were dissected to detect the exact localization of the tumor. Strips of the transitional zone between normal and malignant tissue were sampled. The strips were divided to obtain several samples. Some samples were formalin fixed and then paraffin embedded. Others were fixed and prepared according to the Karnovsky procedure, plastic embedded, and then analyzed by electron microscopy [2].

Sections (5 μm) were cut from the paraffin-emedded tissue stripes, and routinely H&E stained. Immunohistochemistry was performed with mono-

Table 1. Patient data and morphological characteristics of the renal tumors

Patient no.	Age (years)	Sex	Tumor size (cm)	Tumor stage
1	58	F	8	pT 3
2	60	M	9	pT 3
3	54	F	6	pT 2
4	69	M	7.5	pT 3
5	45	F	9	pT 3
6	76	M	10	pT 3
7	71	M	6	pT 3
8	61	M	5.5	pT 2
9	53	M	4.5	pT 2
10	74	F	6	pT 2
11	64	M	3	pT 1
12	71	M	9	pT 3
13	59	F	11	pT 3

Table 2. Specificity, localization, and dilution source of the monoclonal antibodies

Antibody	Specificity	Localization	Dilution	Source
MA-931	Muscle-specific actin	Skeletal, smooth, cardiac muscle	1:200	Enzo
D 33	Desmin	Skeletal, smooth, cardiac muscle	1:100	Dako
KL 1	Cytokeratin (56 kDa)	Epithelial cells	1:400	Dianova
CIV 22	Collagen IV	Basement membrane	1:40	Dako

clonal antibodies against cytokertin, collagen IV, and muscle-specific actin and desmin. The characterisics of the monoclonal antibodies used in this study are presented in Table 2. We performed the alkaline phosphatase–antialkaline phosphatase staining technique; new fuchsin was used as substrate [1]. Slides were counterstained with hematoxylin [6].

Results

Light Microscopy and Immunohistochemistry

All tumors investigated in this study were encapsuled. Each capsule was relatively homogeneous, exhibiting minimal variation in density and thickness only. By light microscopy the capsule was found to consist of layers of collagen fibers separated from each other by long tiny cells, better visible by electron microscopy as outlined below. The capsules of different tumors varied between a few to many hundreds of layers of collagen fibers. Only a few small vessels crossed the capsule. However, some large arteries were found crossing the capsular zone; their elastic tissue was clearly identified by immunostaining.

Compressed remnants of renal cells and tissue were located in the non-malignant tissue area close to the capsule. These compressed normal renal corpuscles, although located in normal renal tissue, exhibited different stages of sclerosis; some tubuli contained protein casts while, the closer to the capsule, other tubuli had almost disappeared, and only single cells or a few connective cellular elements were remaining. In all 13 cases the tumor capsule exhibited strong staining for muscle-specific actin (Fig. 1a). The staining was confined to the cytoplasm of long thin cells layered in a tangential pattern within the capsule. Moreover, the smooth-muscle cells in the media of arteries crossing the capsule were positive with antiactin antibodies. Desmin showed a similar distribution within the tumor capsules, but the staining intensity and density was weaker (Fig. 1b). Weak staining of the extracellular component of the capsule was obtained by anti-collagen VI (Fig. 1c). With anti-cytokeratin antibodies single epithelial cells as remnants of compressed tubuli within the capsule were detected.

Electron Microscopic Findings

In agreement with previous investigations [9], the capsule consisted of numerous layers of flattened, elongated cells separated from each other by collagen fibers, elastic fibers, remnants of renal corpuscles, and tubules in various stages of sclerosis and atrophy (Fig. 2). Most of the flattened cells had typical landmarks of smooth-muscle cells, for example, an elongated, centrally positioned indented nucleus and a discontinuous, deeply stained peripheral rim of cytoplasm. By electron microscopy the cells showed a discontinuous basement

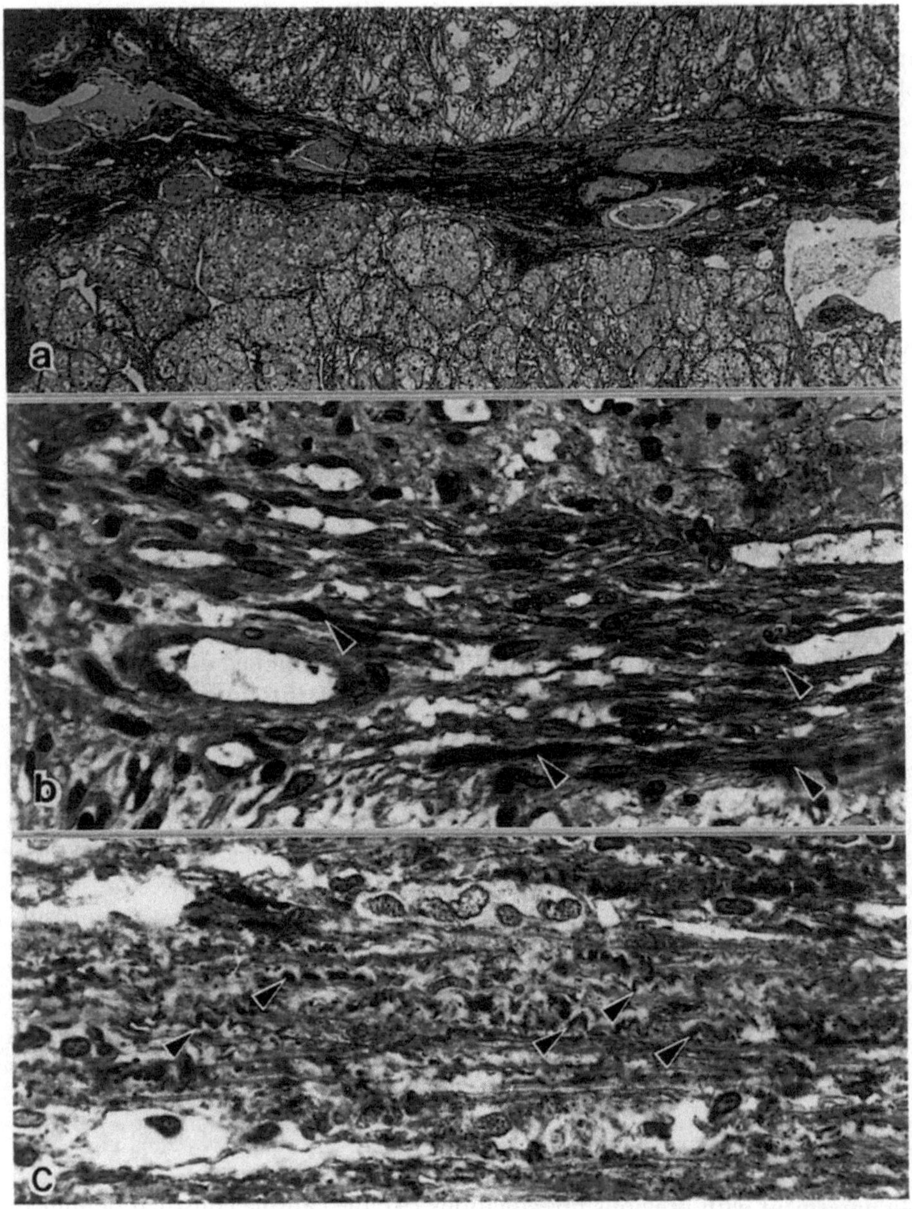

Fig. 1. Immunohistochemical localization of anti-actin (**a**), anti-desmin (**b**), and anti-collagen (**c**) antibodies within the tumor capsule. **a** Tumor capsule, dark cells (smooth-muscle cells) are stained by anti-actin. Within the capsule vessels and remnants of normal renal corpuscles in different stages of sclerosis are found. ×50. **b** Higher magnification (×420) of the same capsule. *Arrowheads*, desmin-positive cells. **c** Basement membrane material and collagen fibers (collagen IV; *arrowheads*). ×420

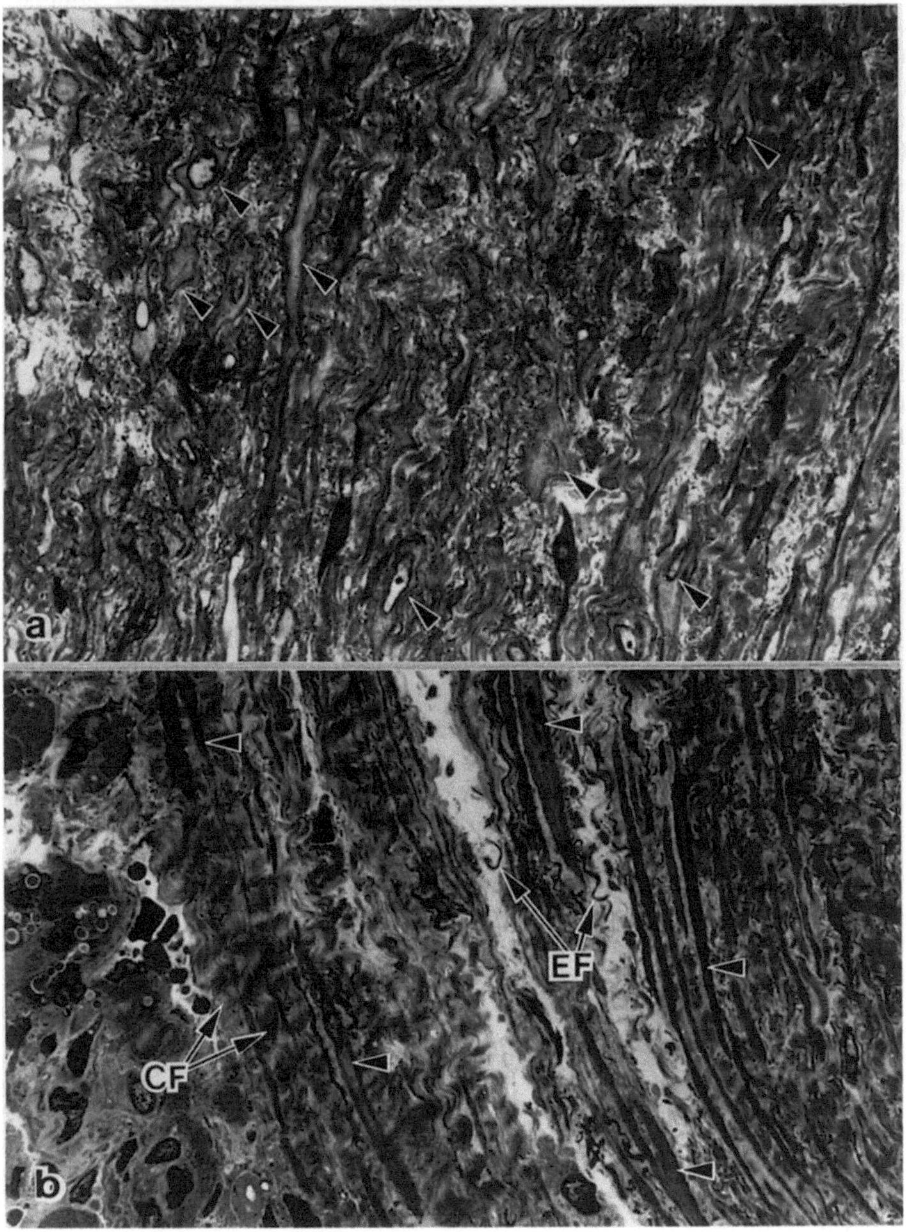

Fig. 2a, b. Sections of plastic-embedded specimens, electron microscopic findings. **a** Outer region of the tumor capsule. *Arrowheads*, some body and tiny processes of the numerous elongated cells with characteristics of smooth-muscle cells. **b** Transitional zone from the capsule to the tumor (*left*). Elongated cells (*arrowheads*), collagen (*CF*), and elastic (*EF*) fibers. ×850 membrane, assemblies of caveolae alternating with dense bodies or plaques along the plasma membrane (Figs. 3, 4). Dense bodies were occasionally scattered inside the cell, among numerous filaments measuring 6 nm in diameter (Fig. 4). The rough endoplasmic reticulum was abundant, especially at the poles of the nucleus. A few small mitochondria and glycogen granules were also seen (Fig. 4). In addition to this largely predominant cell type, a few fibrocytes were scattered throughout the tumoral capsule (Fig. 3). As seen by light microscopy, thick collagen fibers, which were always oriented parallel to the tumoral surface, marked the border of the capsule toward the malignant tissue (Fig. 2b). Between the collagen fibers there were elastic fibers with irregular length (Fig. 2b, 4a). In the extracellular matrix electron microscopy revealed further tubular microfibrils about 12 nm in diameter (Fig. 4b) and assemblies of basement membrane-like material of very different extension (Fig. 3), as well as filamentous structures (presumably proteoglycans) which were connected to the collagen fibrils or lay free in the interfibrillar space (Fig. 4).

Discussion

The tumor capsule is an early-stage phenomenon of RCC. This histomorphological structure of the transitional zone between normal and malignant renal tissue is composed of cells which, due to their immunohistochemical and electron microscopic characteristics, have been described as smooth-muscle cells. These cells are positive for actin and desmin, as known for smooth-muscle cells of the tunica media of arteries [2, 9]. Immunohistochemical findings support the view that the tumor capsule contains contractile cells. As mentioned above, fixation by vascular perfusion of encapsuled RCC is frequently unsuccessful. According to clinical experience, it is rare for the primary tumor of the kidney in metastatic RCC patients to respond to any currently known systemic therapy such as chemotherapy or immunotherapy with cytokines, whereas metastatic lesions exhibit a response rate up to 30% [4, 8]. Our hypothesis is that the increasing tissue pressure of the growing tumor causes the atrophy and sclerosis of the surrounding normal tissue. Within the tumor capsule only remnants of normal parenchymal cells are found, whereas a high number of smooth-muscle cells and collagen as well as elastic fibers are observed. The origin of the smooth-muscle cells, collagen, and elastic fibers is obviously the normal renal tissue.

The tumor capsule resembles a barrier confining the malignant tumor. It is unknown, whether this is an active or passive reaction or process of the normal renal tissue.

A MDP scintigram is routinely used for bone scan to examine patients with malignancies concerning bone metastases, but this technique can also be taken as a parameter to detect the interstitial distribution of drugs within the human kidney. Patients with histologically confirmed RCC normally exhibit a filling defect of the tumor area within the kidney compared to the normal renal tissue

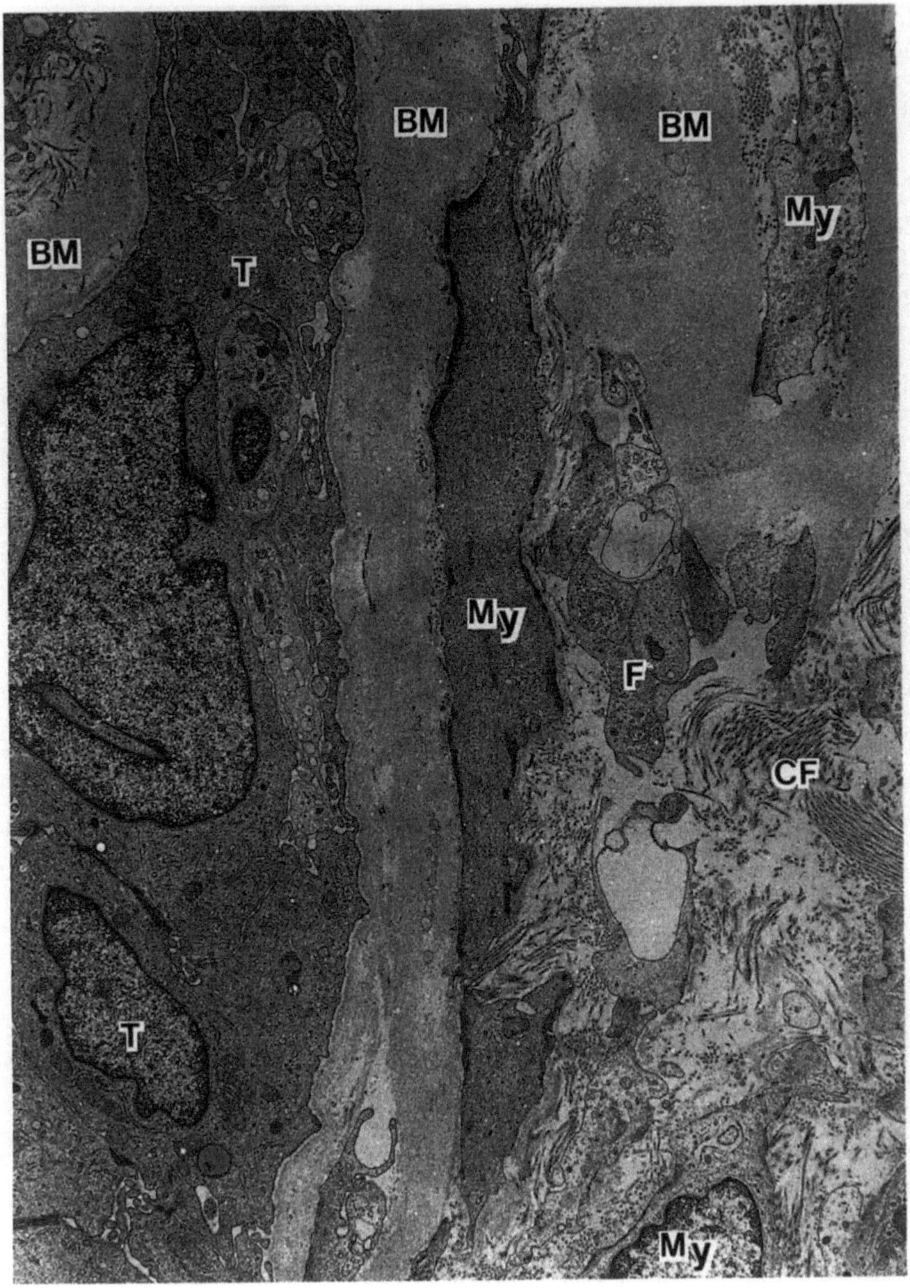

Fig. 3. Electron microscopic specimen. The tumor capsule is composed of remnants of normal renal parenchyma: tubule cells (*T*), smooth-muscle cells (*My*), fibroblasts (*F*), collagen fibers (*CF*), and basement membrane material (*BM*). ×16000

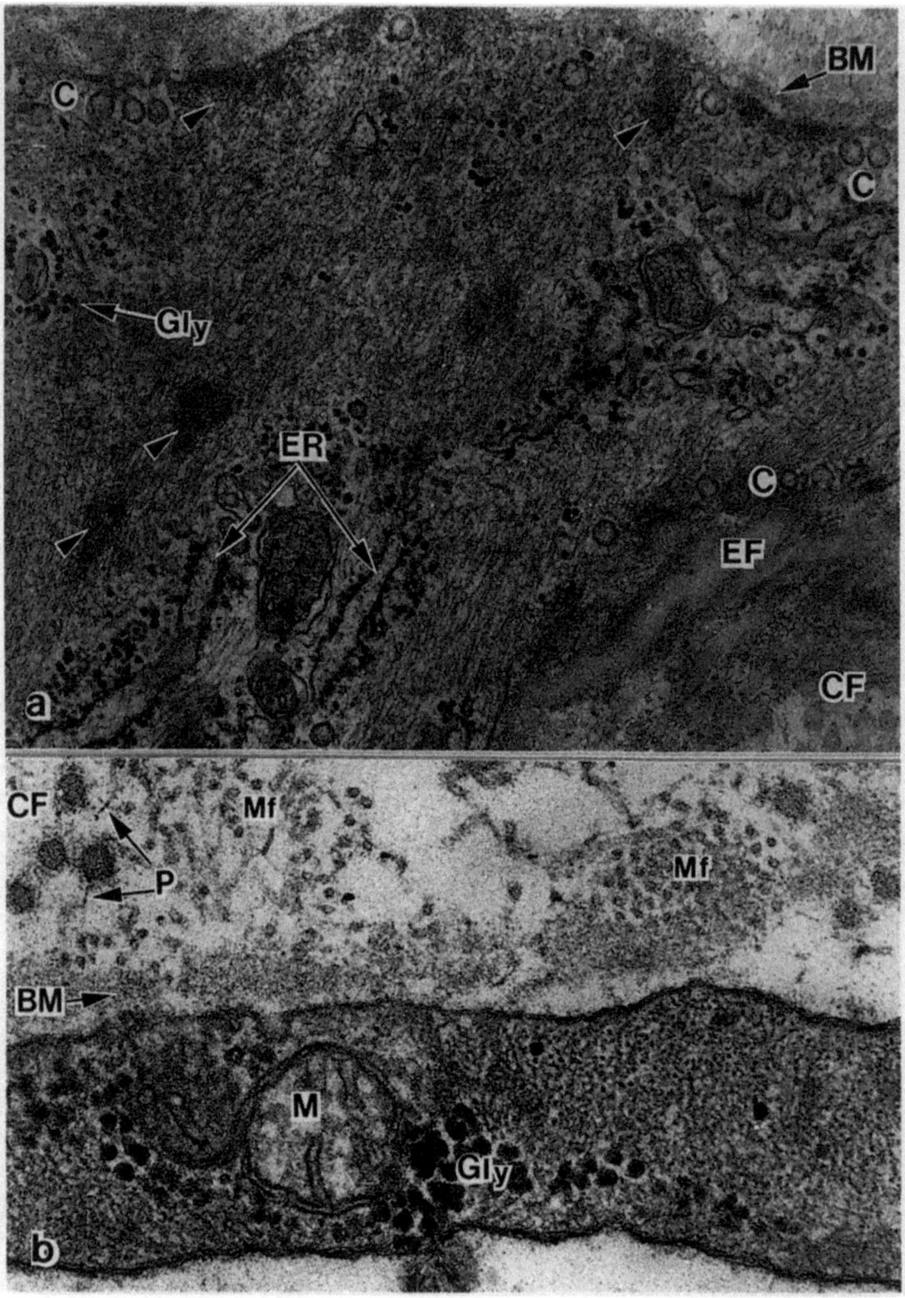

Fig. 4a, b. Electron microscopic specimen. Smooth-muscle cell in longitudinal (**a**) and in cross-section (**b**). **a** Filaments, dense bodies (some indicated by *arrowheads*), caveolae (*C*), mitochondria, glycogen granules (*Gly*), rough-surfaced endoplasmic reticulum (*ER*), and discontinuous basement membrane (*BM*). In the extracellular matrix, collagen (*CF*) and elastic fibrils (*EF*). **b** Filaments, mitochondria (*M*), glycogen particles (*Gly*), basement membrane (*BM*), tubular microfibrils (*MF*), collagen fibrils (*CF*) with associated thin filaments presumably of proteoglycans (*P*). **a** × 60 000. **b** × 80 000

[8]. All these findings indicate that the malignant renal tissue may have a higher tissue pressure compared to normal renal tissue, obviously caused by the increased growth rate [10].

The tumor capsule in the function of a barrier between normal and malignant tissue and the increased tissue pressure of the tumor may both cause the decreased interstitial substance or drug concentration within the tumor compared to the surrounding normal renal tissue or to the tissue of other organs. This may be one of the main reasons that the local tumor within the kidney of metastatic RCC patients shows nearly no response to any known systemic treatment such as chemotherapy or immunotherapy, whereas metastatic lesions (in other organs, e.g., in the lungs) exhibit a therapeutic response rate up to 30% and more [4, 11].

References

1. Cordell JL, Falini B, Erber NW, Ghosh AK, Abdulaziz Z, Mac-Donald S, Pulford KAF, Stein H, Mason DY (1984) Immunoenzymatic labeling of monoclonal antibodies using immune complexes of alkaline phosphatase and monoclonal antialkaline phosphatase (APAAP complexes). J Histochem Cytochem 32: 219–229
2. Karnovsky MJ (1971) Use of ferrocyanide-reduced osmium tetroxide in electron microscopy. Abstracts of the American Society of Cell Biology, New Orleans, p 146
3. de Kernion JB (1986) Renal tumors. In: Walsh PC, Gittes RF, Perlmutter AD, Stamey TA (eds) Campbell's urology, vol 2. Saunders, Philadelphia, pp 1297–1342
4. Kirchner H, de Riese W, Allhoff E, Poliwoda H, Atzpodien J (1991) Immunotherapy of advanced renal cell cancer using subcutaneous recombinant interleukin-2 and interferon-alpha. World J Urol 9: 219–222
5. Kuehn K, Panzer J, Luciano L, Reale E (1985) Identification of proteoglycans in the rat and human glomerular basement membrane. In: Lubec G, Hudson BG (eds) Glomerular basement membrane. Libbey, London, pp 17–20
6. Lelle RJ, Heidenreich W, Stauch G, Gerdes J (1987) The correlation of growth fractions with histologic grading and lymph node status in human mammary carcinoma. Cancer 59: 83–88
7. Lubarsch O (1925) Die destruierenden Nierengewaechse. In: Henke F, Lubarsch O (eds) Handbuch der speziellen pathologischen Anatomie und Histologie. Springer, Berlin, p 636
8. de Riese W, Allhoff EP (1991) Einsatz von Biological Response Modifiers in der Behandlung des metastasierten Nierenzellkarzinoms; Review der klinischen Daten. In: de Riese W, Allhoff EP, Schuth J, Jonas U (eds) Das metastasierte Nierenzellkarzinom, Klinik und therapeutische Aspekte. Springer, Berlin Heidelberg New York, pp 25–41
9. de Riese W, Reale E (1991) The capsule of the renal cell carcinoma contains modified smooth muscle cells. J Submicrosc Cytol Pathol 23(2): 237–244
10. de Riese W, Allhoff E, Werner M, Atzpodien J, Kirchner H, Stief CG, Djamilian M, Schlick R, Jonas U (1991) Proliferative behaviour and cytogenetic changes in human renal cell carcinoma (RCC). World J Urol 9: 79–85
11. Yagoda A (1992) Cytotoxic chemotherapy trials between 1983 and 1990 for advanced renal cell carcinoma. In: Staehler G, Pomer S (eds) Basic and clinical research on renal cell carcinoma. Springer, Berlin Heidelberg New York, pp 71–78

Interleukin-2 Therapy: Report on 129 Patients and Three Different Schedules

S. NÉGRIER[1], A. MERCATELLO[2], B. CORONEL[2], F. LANIER[1], M.O. HEILMANN[2], Y. MERROUCHE[1], M. BRET[2], J.Y. BLAY[1], C. LASSET[1], M. FAVROT[1], J.F. MOSKOVTCHENKO[2], and T. PHILIP[1]

Approximately one-half of patients with renal carcinoma develop metastases, and these have a median survival of 8 months [6, 11, 12]. Metastatic renal cancer has been considered for the past 20 years as a tumor resistant to conventional therapies, and great hopes have therefore been placed on the potential role of immunotherapy in this disease. Since 1984 interleukin-2 (IL-2) has been widely used in oncology and has been registered as a drug for use in metastatic renal cell carcinoma (MRCC) treatment in Europe and the United States [8, 12]. However, although IL-2 is now generally accepted as integral in the management of MRCC, its optimal administration is still a matter of debate. Table 1 reports the results of trials using IL-2 in the treatment of metastatic renal carcinoma.

We report here our own experience with immunotherapy in metastatic renal carcinoma. Between October 1987 and August 1991, 181 patients were referred to our Institute. Of these, 129 underwent IL-2 therapy while 52 were excluded according to the exclusion criteria. Different successive protocols were used, defining three distinct groups of patients (Table 2). The first group ($n = 50$), as part of a European multicenter trial, received continuous infusion of IL-2 according to the schedule of West et al. [16] – with and without lymphokine-activated killer cells (LAK cells). The second group ($n = 37$) were treated according to a combined schedule of 5-day subcutaneous interferon (IFN) at 20×10^6 U/day and, after a 2-day break, 5-day intravenous treatment with IL-2 (24×10^6 IU/m^2 three times per day) and IFN (5×10^6 U/m^2 three times per day) repeated after a 6-day rest. During the last 5 days of treatment LAK cells were reinjected together with the therapy. Finally, a cohort of patients ($n = 35$) received the combined subcutaneous schedule of Atzpodien et al. [1, 2] (ten patients were treated at Bordeaux).

None of these patients had previously undergone any systemic therapy. Table 3 shows the grade 4 (World Health Organization) toxic events observed with each therapy regimen. Although the subcutaneous schedule was not

[1] Department of Medical Oncology and Biostatistic Unit, Centre Léon BERARD, 28 rue Laënnec, F-69373 Lyon, Cédex 08, France
[2] Intensive Care Unit, Hôpital Edouard HERRIOT, Pavillon P, place d'Arsonval, F-69008 Lyon, France

Table 1. Summary of major IL-2 therapeutic studies in metastatic renal carcinoma

Reference	*n*	Regimen	Response		
			CR	PR	CR + PR (%)
Rosenberg et al. [14]	54	IL-2 (hdb)	4	8	22
Rosenberg et al. [14]	72	IL-2 + LAK (hdb)	8	17	35
Rosenberg et al. [13]	46	IL-2 + IFN (hdb)	4	11	32
West [16]	23	IL-2 + LAK (ci)	2	5	30
Négrier et al. [8]	51	IL-2 + LAK (ci)	5	9	27
Négrier et al. [8]	32	IL-2 (ci)	2	4	197
Atzpodien et al. [2]	34	IL-2 + IFN (sc)	4	6	29

hdb, High-dose bolus; ci, continuous infusion; sc, subcutaneous; CR, complete response; PR, partial response.

Table 2. Different IL-2 schedules used at Lyon

Regimen	*n*	Response		
		CR	PR	CR + PR (%)
IL-2 + LAK (ci)	20	0	4	18
IL-2 (ci)	27	2	3	18
IL-2 + IFN + LAK (hdb)	34	2	6	24
IL-2 + IFN (sc)	34	1	6	20

ci, Continuous infusion; hdb, high-dose bolus; sc, subcutaneous; CR, complete response; PR, partial response.

Table 3. Grade 4 (WHO) toxicity observed in IL-2 treatment regimen at Lyon

	IL-2 or IL-2 + LAK (intravenous continuous infusion) (*n* = 50)	IL-2 + IFN + LAK (intravenous bolus dose) (*n* = 37)	IL-2 + IFN (subcutaneous low doses) (*n* = 35)
Adverse events	1 respiratory distress (pneumothorax)	1 toxic death (myocardiopathy)	No grade 4 toxicity
	1 respiratory distress (IL-2 + tumor progression)	1 nonfatal cardiac arrest	
		1 major hypotension	
	1 toxic death (cardiac)	1 acute renal failure requiring dialysis	
Percentage	6%	11%	0%

responsible for any life-threatening toxicity, general symptoms were always present, and most patients complained about the duration of this schedule and the associated chronicity of fever, fatigue, and anorexia. Notably, in this series a cohort of 25 patients aged over 65 years were treated with continuous infusion of IL-2, as has been previously reported [9]. Toxicity was manifested as before but with additional cardiac toxicity. Changes in cardiac rhythm occurred in 44% of patients and were clearly involved in one toxic death.

Response was comparable to that reported by others. It was found that the most intensive schedule gave the highest response rate. Furthermore, the combination of IL-2 and IFN did not lead to any dramatic augmentation in the number of responders. The median duration of complete response was 20 months. Figure 1 shows an example of complete remission in a patient who is still in good health 3 years after treatment.

As shown in Figs. 2 and 3, survival was analyzed and compared to our historical control group of 129 patients considered for survival analysis. Of these, 122 have already received IL-2 as first-line therapy while 7 who had previously undergone IFN therapy elsewhere were treated with IL-2 plus tumor necrosis factor as second-line of treatment (data previously reported [10]). The most important conclusion is that immunotherapy with IL-2 is not applicable to all patients but leads to the exclusion of a group of patients with a limited survival. Nevertheless, as shown in Figure 3, there is a significant difference between the historical control group and all the patients treated subsequently at Lyon (log rank 21.5).

Of greatest importance in these results is that – irrespective of the dose schedule and the IL-2 in combination with IFN – response rates were approximately 25% [8, 13, 15, 16]. Very little is known about the mechanisms underlying IL-2 induced tumor regression. During the past 5 years different hypotheses have been considered, such as the changes in immune phenotypes of circulating lymphocytes [7], although these findings have not been confirmed in more comprehensive studies [13, 16]. The role of HLA antigen expression on tumor cells has also been reported but has not been confirmed as yet [5]. More recently, the presence of sustained endogenous production of tumor necrosis factor after cessation of IL-2 therapy [3] and the presence of serum interleukin-6 prior to the therapy appeared as important prognostic factors in patients undergoing IL-2 therapy [4]. The mechanisms involved in the anticancer activity of IL-2 are complex and probably depend on immune factors as well as tumor determinants. The understanding of these mechanisms will be an important challenge for immuno-oncologists for the next few years.

Clinicians can, however, in a more empirical fashion, attempt to improve the results of current IL-2 therapy in MRCC. The results of our survival study emphasize that, even if the patients receiving a specific treatment have been selected, and although only 20% respond to therapy, overall survival is improved. The exact role of IL-2 therapy in this respect is unknown since this phenomenon could be a function of improved general management, including

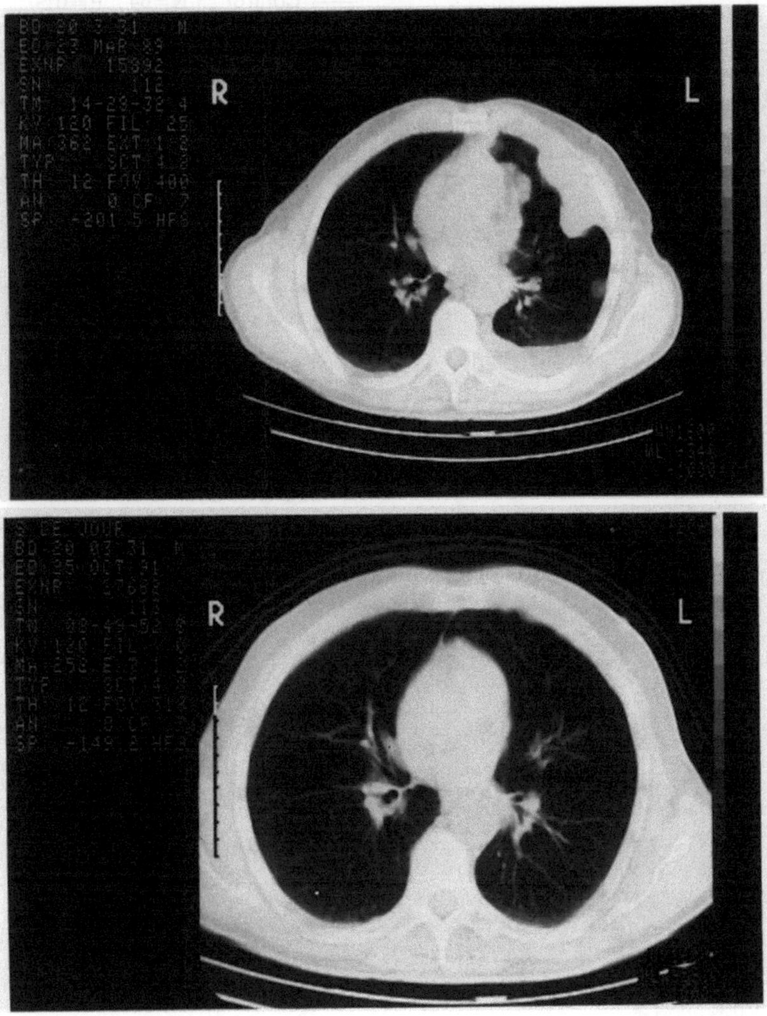

a

b

Fig. 1a, b. Computed tomography showing pericardic and pleural metastases with contiguous involvement of the rib in a patient with MRCC. **a** Before treatment. **b** After treatment

palliative support. Until now, no comparative prospective study investigating survival gain with IL-2 therapy has been carried out. On the other hand, for ethical reasons, a randomized trial IL-2 versus placebo does not appear feasible. Therefore, a large multicenter randomized study is now being organized in France. The aim of this study is to evaluate response and survival rates of patients with MRCC receiving three different regimes – intravenous IL-2,

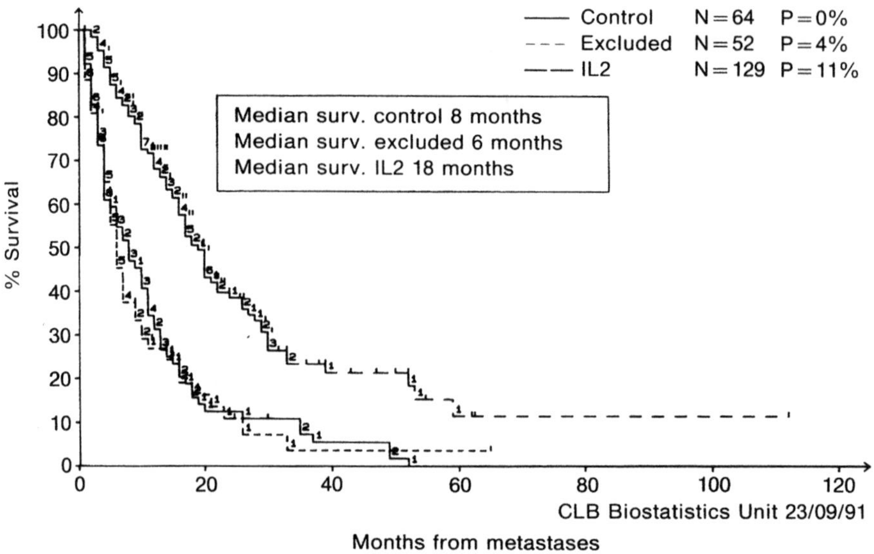

Fig. 2. Survival of the three cohorts of patients at Lyon

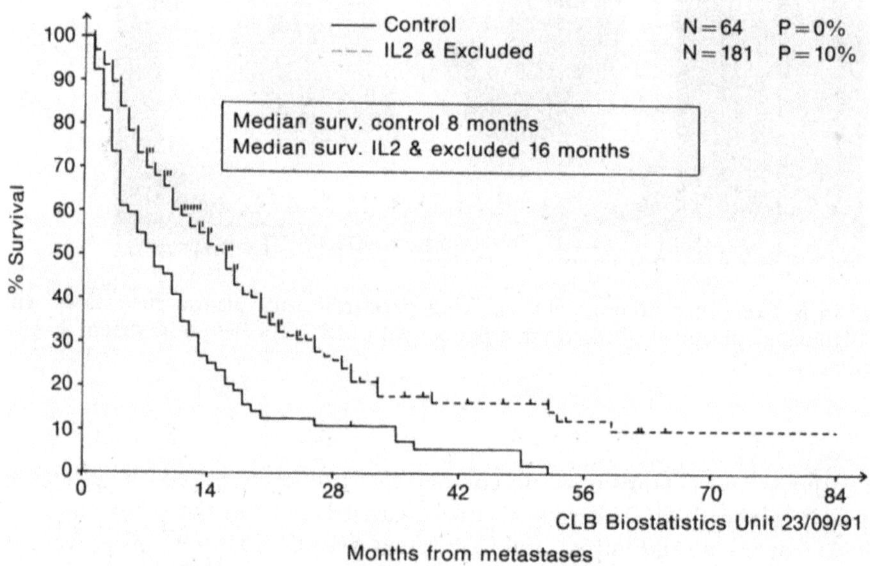

Fig. 3. Survivals of Lyon's historical control group versus IL-2 treated patients and excluded patients

subcutaneous IFN, and the combination of IL-2 and IFN – according to their prognosis factors.

In conclusion, IL-2 is active in MRCC and should be proposed for a maximum number of patients. However, several important questions remain regarding the biological mechanisms of tumor regression as well as the most appropriate schedule of IL-2 therapy.

Acknowledgements. Supported by the Association de Recherche Contre le Cancer (1987–1990) and Ligue Nationale Contre le Cancer (1991–1992).

References

1. Atzpodien J, Körfer A, Franks CR, Poliwoda H, Kinchner H (1990) Home therapy with recombinant interleukin-2 and interferon alpha in advanced malignancies. Lancet 335: 1509–1512
2. Atzpodien J, Körfer A, Menzel T, Poliwoda H, Kirchner H (1991) (abstract). Proc Am Soc Clin Oncol 10: 571
3. Blay JY, Favrot MC, Négrier S et al. (1990) Correlation between clinical response to interleukin-2 and sustained production of TNF. Cancer Res 50: 2371–2374
4. Blay JY, Négrier S, Combaret V et al. (1992) Serum level of interleukin-6 as a prognostic factor in metastatic renal cell carcinoma. Cancer Res 52: 3317–3322
5. Cohen PJ, Lotze MT, Roberts JR, Rosenberg SA, Jaffe ES (1987) The immunopathology of sequential tumor biopsies in patients treated with interleukin-2: correlations of response with T cell infiltration and HLA DR expression. Am J Pathol 129: 208–216
6. De Forges A, Rey A, Klinik A, Ghosn M, Kramar A, Droz JP (1988) Prognostic factors of adult metastatic renal carcinoma: a multivariate analysis. Semin Surg Oncol 4: 149–154
7. Favrot MC, Combaret V, Négrier S et al. (1990) Functional and immunophenotypic modifications induced by interleukin-2 did not predict the response to therapy in patients with metastatic renal carcinoma. J Biol Response Mod 9: 167–177
8. Négrier S, Philip T, Stoter G et al. (1989) Interleukin-2 with or without LAK cells in metastatic renal cell carcinoma; a report of an European multicentric study. Eur J Cancer Clin Oncol 25: S1–S28
9. Négrier S, Mercatello A, Bret M et al. (1992) Intravenous interleukin-2 in patients over 65 with metastatic renal carcinoma. Br J Cancer 65: 723–726
10. Négrier MS, Pourreau CN, Palmer P et al. (1992) Phase I trial of recombinant interleukin-2 followed by recombinant tumor necrosis factor in patients with metastatic cancer. J Immun 11: 93–102
11. Philip T, Mercatello A, Négrier S et al. (1989) Interleukin-2 with or without LAK cells in metastatic renal cell carcinoma: the Lyon first year experience on 20 patients. Cancer Treat Rev 16: 91–104
12. Rosenberg SA, Lotze MT, Muul LM et al. (1987) A progress report on the treatment of 157 patients with advanced cancer using lymphokine activated killer cells and interleukin-2 or high dose interleukin-2 alone. New Engl J Med 316: 889–897
13. Rosenberg SA, Lotze MT, Young JC et al. (1989) Combination therapy with interleukin-2 and alpha-interferon for the treatment of patients with advanced cancer. J Clin Oncol 7: 863–874
14. Rosenberg SA, Lotze MT, Young JC et al. (1989) Experience with the use of high

dose interleukin-2 in the treatment of 652 patients with cancer. Ann Surg 210: 474–485
15. West WH (1989) Continuous infusion recombinant interleukin-2 in adoptive cellular therapy of renal carcinoma and other malignancies. Cancer Treat Rev 16: 83–89
16. West WH, Tauer KW, Yannelli JR et al. (1987) Constant infusion recombinant interleukin-2 in adoptive immunotherapy of advanced cancer. New Engl J Med 316: 898–905

Response According to Site of Metastases in Patients with Metastatic RCC (Renal Cell Carcinoma) During Treatment with Interferon Alpha in Combination with 5-Fluorouracil

A.J.W. GOLDSCHMIDT[1] and U.W. TUNN[2]

We present our preliminary results. Of 30 patients with M_1 renal cell carcinoma, 21 were included in our prospective controlled pilot study until March 14, 1992. These 21 patients were evaluated for efficacy in the treatment with recombinant interferon alfa-2b in combination with 5-fluorouracil (5-FU).

The clinical response according to the WHO criteria has been studied to determine whether it is associated with the metastases' site and biological behavior. The important factors were:

1. Definite M_1 status
2. Prior nephrectomy
3. Karnofsky-index greater or equal 70%. Patients with another malignoma, CNS metastases, or previous chemo-, cytokine, or radiation therapy were excluded from the study.

Interferon alfa-2b was given at a dose of 5 MIU subcutaneously days 1–5 every week for 14 weeks. 5-FU was given at a dose of 500 mg/m^2 days 1–5 in weeks 2, 6, 10, and 14. For the detailed regimen, see Fig. 1.

The mean Karnofsky performance status fell during the 14 weeks of therapy from 88.7% to 81.1%, and the mean body weight from 76.7 kg to 74.2 kg. Side effects (Table 1) and laboratory investigations showed no unexpected characteristics. Most apparent were the reversible changes of platelets, leukocytes, serum alkaline phosphatase, and gamma glutamate transaminase. The therapy was well tolerated.

During the 14 weeks the combination therapy led to objective remissions (complete and partial) in 24% ($n = 5$) of patients and to a stable disease in 33% ($n = 7$). The sites of metastases of the responders were in three cases the lung, in one case the lung in combination with positive lymph nodes, and only in one further case bone (solitary, thoracic vertebra 9). Three patients with stable

[1] Städtische Kliniken Offenbach, Urologische Klinik, Akademisches Lehrkrankenhaus der Universität Frankfurt/Main, and Abteilung Medizinische Informatik und Biometrie, Starkenburgring 66, D-63069 Offenbach, Germany
[2] Städtische Kliniken Offenbach, Urologische Klinik, Akademisches Lehrkrankenhaus der Universität Frankfurt/Main, Starkenburgring 66, D-63069 Offenbach, Germany

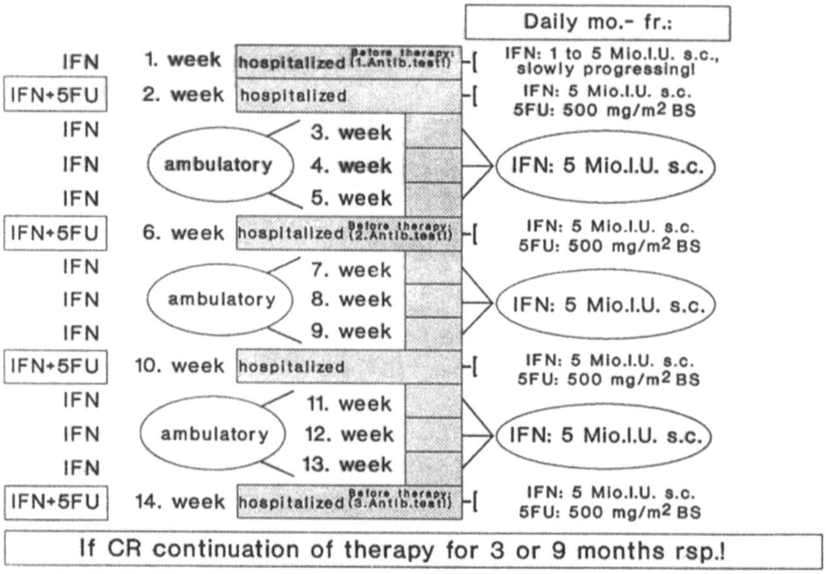

Fig. 1. Detailed therapeutic regimen. Interferon alfa-2b and 5-fluorouracil in M_1-renal cell carcinoma. *Hospitalized* means performed in our hospital; *ambulatory* means therapy provided by a privately practicing urologist or at an outpatient ambulatory urological practice

Table 1. Side effects of interferon alpha therapy ($n = 19$)

Side effects	Patients	
	(n)	(%)
Weakness	9	47.4
Nausea	9	47.4
Loss of vitality	7	36.8
Inappetence	5	26.3
Slight dyspnea	3	15.8
Myelosuppression G II	3	15.8
Pruritus	2	10.5
Fever	1	5.2
Stomatitis	1	5.2
Dysphagia	1	5.2
Loss of weight	1	5.2
Diarrhea	1	5.2

disease had lung and four had bone metastases. The site of metastases of the nonresponders (43%, $n = 9$) was in five cases the lung and in four cases bones. Only in the nonresponder group have there been two RCC-related deaths (in weeks 2 and 26). One of these patients had lung and the other bone metastases.

There is obviously a clear trend for lung and soft tissue metastases to respond to therapy (4 of 12 = 33%), while bone metastases do not or only poorly respond (1 of 9 = 8%). The site of metastases remains the most important prognosticator for response to therapy with interferon alfa-2b in combination with 5-FU.

II Basic Research

Molecular Mapping of the Human 3p Region

E.R. Zabarovsky[1,2], V.I. Kashuba[1], Z. Marcsek[3], E.S. Pokrovskaya[1], V.Zabarovska[1], I. Kholodnyuk[1], R. Erlandsson[1], J. Sumegi[4], G. Winberg[1], L.L. Kisselev[2], and G. Klein[1]

Introduction

The aim of this study is to identify the gene(s) on the short arm of human chromosome 3, the loss of which contributes to the occurrence of kidney carcinoma and other solid tumors. The critical role of aberrations detected on the short arm of chromosome 3 have been suggested by recent cytogenetic and molecular studies with restriction fragment length polymorphism in relation to the development of renal cell carcinoma [6, 7], von Hippel Lindau disease [13], lung cancer [9], and breast cancer [3]. The majority of the RCC tumors can be characterized cytogenetically by deletions of the short arm of chromosome 3 from 3p13 to 3pter [7]. Restriction fragment length polymorphism analysis of tumor-derived DNA have revealed allelic losses of known polymorphic DNA markers localized to various parts of 3p, suggesting the involvement of a tumor suppressor gene, probably near the D3F15S2 marker (3p21), in the origin and/or evolution of renal cell carcinoma [6]. The search for a tumor suppressor gene in the affected region, however, is hampered by the size of the chromosomal segment involved (minimal estimation is 40 Mbp) along the approximately 100 Mbp sized short arm of chromosome 3 [8]. Large areas exist from which no unique sequences are available.

The gap between the resolution of cytogenetic and conventional molecular methods has been successfully bridged by the use of long-range mapping and cloning techniques [2, 12]. One of our approaches for the isolation of the gene(s) whose absence contribute to the development of renal cell carcinoma is based on long-range mapping which includes the use of jumping and linking libraries (Fig. 1). The basic principle of the jumping method is to clone only the ends of large DNA fragments rather than continuous DNA. Internal DNA regions are deleted by biochemical techniques. Although several alternative procedures

[1] Department of Tumor Biology, Karolinska Institutet, Box 60400, S-10401 Stockholm, Sweden
[2] Engelhardt Institute of Molecular Biology, Moscow, Russia
[3] JRO Hungarian Academy of Science and Semmelweis University Medical School, Budapest, Hungary
[4] Department of Pathology and Microbiology, University of Nebraska Medical Center, Omaha, NE, USA

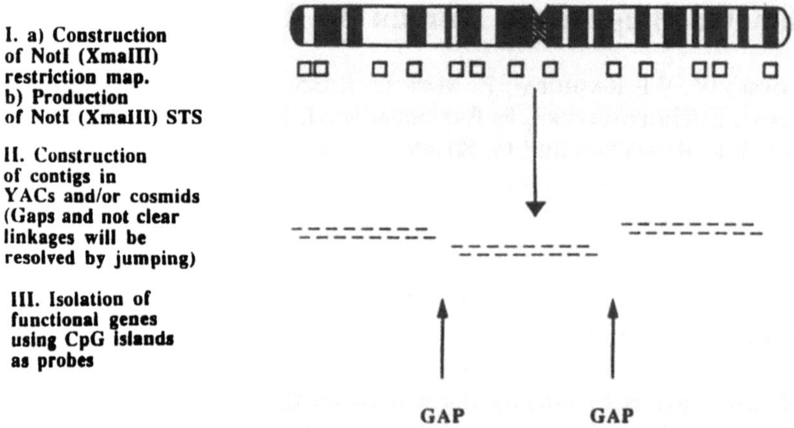

Fig. 1. General strategy of mapping

have been described for construction of linking and jumping libraries [5, 11, 14] all of them have limitations. To make a chromosome jumping library one needs to package a huge amount of vector and to use the *supF* marker with all its disadvantages [2, 12, 17]. These troubles make the use of jumping libraries uncomfortable although construction of such libraries was suggested quite a long time ago [2, 12]. Jumping libraries are usually constructed [2, 12] by the following process. High molecular weight DNA is isolated without mechanical treatment. After cell lysis in low-melting agarose the DNA is either completely or partially digested with a restriction enzyme. Then the DNA in very low concentration and in the presence of a plasmid containing a marker (*supF* gene) is circularized by T4 ligase, trapping the *supF* gene which acts as a marker to detect clones which comprise the ends of a long fragment. The large circular molecules are digested with another enzyme (which has no recognition site in the plasmid) into small fragments, each of which is cloned in a vector phage carrying amber mutations. The ligation mixture is packaged in vitro to form viable phage particles, and bacteria are transfected. Recombinant phages containing the plasmid with two terminal fragments are detected in selective *Escherichia coli* strains lacking the suppressor gene. This procedure yields the jumping library, i.e., a library that includes the terminal parts of the large DNA fragments.

This technique for construction of jumping libraries have several drawbacks. [2, 12, 17]. The vectors used in these experiments are not so convenient, and their cloning capacity is limited to 12 kbp, greatly reducing the representativity of the libraries. Another disadvantage is that only 0.1%–1% of the packaged DNA can represent jumping molecules. This results in the packaging of huge amounts (40–150 μg) of ligation mixture into lambda phage particles. Also the use of *supF* marker creates many problems. It is difficult to predict and find the optimal ratio of genomic DNA to marker. Moreover, because *supF* marker is used in excess. it may block both ends of the same genomic fragment, decreasing the efficiency if the circularization and increasing the possibility of ligation to other DNA fragments, intermolecular ligation frequently occurs. False jumping clones may arise where the two parts of a "jumping" clone represent fragments from different chromosomes. Illegitimate ligation of *supF* into the vector also may generate viable phages without genomic insert. The *supF* function is dependent on its environment. The suppressor-dependent vectors may revert to suppressor-independent ones, although some of the vectors used are multiple amber mutants, which lower the likelihood for such events.

The construction of a linking library, for example, the library of cloned genomic DNA fragments which contain internal sites for rare cutting enzymes, can be performed by different ways [5, 11, 14], but one of the most popular and original methods is similar to that described above and includes the use of *supF* marker, with all its disadvantages [12]. The importance of the jumping and linking libraries usable for many purposes in molecular biology prompted us to develop new lambda vectors and new procedures for construction of linking and jumping libraries.

Construction of New Vectors

A new generation of cloning vectors have been constructed ([15, 16], Table 1). These can be classified either according to their properties or according to the purpose for which they were constructed (as genomic, jumping-linking, or cDNA libraries). The new vectors include: regular lambda phages (SK4, SK6), phasmids (SK2, SK2A), hyphages-phages M13 with the *cos* region of phage

Table 1. Main characteristics of new vectors

Vector	Type of vector	Construction of libraries		
		Genomic	cDNA	Jumping/linking
MC18, MC19	Hyphage	+	+ −	−
SK2A	Phasmid	−	+	−
λSK3, λSK5	λ phage	+	−	−
λSK4, λSK6	λ phage	+	−	+
λSK9, λSK10	Diphasmid, I	+	−	+
λSK11	λ phage	−	+	−
λSK12	Diphasmid, I	−	+	−
λSK15, λSK16	Diphasmid, I	−	+	+
λSK17	Diphasmid, I	−	+	+
λSK18	Diphasmid, II	+	−	−
λSK20, λSK21	Diphasmid, I	+	−	−
λSK22	Diphasmid, I	+	−	+
λSK23, λSK24	Diphasmid, I	+	−	+
λSK25	Diphasmid, I	+	−	+
λSK27	Diphasmid, I	− +	−	+
λSK28	Diphasmid, I	−	+	+
λSK40	Diphasmid, I	+	−	−
λSK41	Diphasmid, I	+	−	+

lambda (MC18, MC19), diphasmids, (i.e., vectors which can exist as plasmids and can be packaged to form lambda or M13 phage particles). The diphasmids are either incapable of lytic growth (SK18) or competent to replicate as lambda phages (SK27, SK28, SK40, SK41, etc). These vectors open new possibilities for gene cloning and analysis.

New Approach for Jumping and Linking Library Construction

The main idea of our approach is to use the same procedure to construct both linking (Fig. 2B) and jumping (Fig. 2A, B) libraries [15–17]. Briefly, the construction of linking and jumping libraries is performed as follows. To construct linking libraries (Fig. 2B) the genomic DNA is digested with *Bam*HI or *Eco*RI, and the DNA is self-ligated at a very low concentration to yield circular molecules as the main product. To eliminate any linear molecules the sticky ends are partly filled-in by the Klenow fragment in the presence of dATP and dGTP. Since the Klenow fragment also has exonuclease activity, all free *Bam*HI sticky ends as well as ends generated upon random DNA breakdown are neutralized, making them unavailable for ligation. The DNA is then cleaved with a restriction enzyme having a rarely occurring recognition sequence (*Not*I, *Sal*I, *Xho*I, *Xma*III) and ligated to lambda SK17 and lambda SK22 "arms." The ligation product is packaged in vitro into phage lambda particles. The phage particles are used to infect *E. coli* cells in which only recombinant phages can grow. The construction of *Not*I jumping libraries [17] starts with complete *Not*I digestion of DNA in agarose blocks and is followed by the self-ligation at very low DNA concentration (Fig. 2A). Other steps are exactly the same as those used for the construction of linking libraries.

Using these procedures, we have constructed chromosome 3 specific and total human linking libraries for *Not*I, *Sal*I, *Xho*I, and *Xma*III. DNA was isolated from the human microcell/mouse hybrid cell line MCH903.1, carrying a complete human chromosome 3 [15], MCH924.4, containing human chromosome 3 with interstitial deletion of the region 3p13–p22 (unpublished results) and from DNA of the human lymphoblastoid cell line CBMI-Ral-STO (4, Table 2). About 3%–5% of the clones isolated from the microcell hybrid cell lines hybridized to total human DNA. All of our libraries can be considered very representative ones, taking into account that the whole human genome contains about 3000 *Not*I sites and about 30 000 *Xma*III, *Sal*I, or *Xho*I sites and the human chromosome 3 about 10% of them. The size of the inserted DNA varies between 3 and 23 kbp, which is sufficient to allow the identification of human clones on the basis of their content of human repetitive sequences. Several libraries and also individual clones have been transferred into plasmid form to simplify their handling. From the human chromosome 3 specific libraries plasmid clones have been selected and filtergrids of ordered clones prepared: grid no. 1, *Not*I linking, specific for whole chromosome 3 (DNA was from MCH903.1; 900 clones were put on the grid); grid no. 2, *Not*I linking, specific for

Table 2. General characteristics of linking and jumping libraries

Library no.	Name of library	Source of DNA	Specificity	Type	Enzymes	Lambda vector	No. of i.r.
1	NLM	MCH903.1	Total chr. 3	Linking	*Not*I/*Bam*HI	SK17&22	0.65 × 105
2	NL1	MCH903.1	Total chr. 3	Linking	*Not*I/*Bam*HI	SK17	1 × 105
3	NL2	MCH903.1	Total chr. 3	Linking	*Not*I/*Bam*HI	SK22	0.65 × 105
4	BSL	MCH903.1	Total chr. 3	Linking	*Sal*I/*Bam*HI	SK17&22	1.5 × 106
5	BCL	MCH903.1	Total chr. 3	Linking	*Xho*I/*Bam*HI	SK17&22	1.8 × 106
6	BXL	MCH903.1	Total chr. 3	Linking	*Xam*III/*Bam*HI	SK4,17&22	0.8 × 106
7	924	MCH924.4	del (3p13–22)	Linking	*Not*I/*Bam*HI	SK17&22	1 × 105
8	HL-NB	CBMI-RaI-STO	Total human	Linking	*Not*I/*Bam*HI	SK4,17&22	5.5 × 105
9	HL-NR	CBMI-RaI-STO	Total human	Linking	*Not*I/*Eco*RI	SK4,17&22	5.1 × 105
10	NRL	MCH903.1	Total chr. 3	Linking	*Not*I/*Eco*RI	SK17	0.7 × 105
11	HL-XB	CBMI-RaI-STO	Total human	Linking	*Xho*I/*Bam*HI	SK4,17&22	1 × 106
12	HL-XR	CBMI-RaI-STO	Total human	Linking	*Xho*I/*Eco*RI	SK4,17&22	1 × 106
13	j21,j22	CBMI-RaI-STO	Total human	Jumping	*Not*I/*Bam*HI	SK17&22	2.2 × 105
14	j31,j32	MCH903.1	Total chr. 3	Jumping	*Not*I/*Bam*HI	SK17&22	5 × 105

chromosome 3 with 3p13–p22 deleted region (DNA from MCH924.4; 230 clones); and grid no. 3, *Not*I jumping, specific for whole chromosome 3 (DNA was from MCH903.1; 610 clones). An additional grid containing 1200 chromosome 3 specific *Not*I linking clones in lambda form was also constructed.

The major features of our protocol are as follows. For construction of the *Not*I jumping and linking libraries two or three vectors are used simultaneously. The properties of these vectors were optimized for this purpose. The lambda arms cannot produce viable phages without an insert; the combined cloning capacity of the three vectors is between 0.2 and 24 kbp – compared to a vector capacity of only 0–12 kbp in some schemes [2, 12] and 9–24 kbp in others [2, 12]. Thus, our vectors help to increase representativity and lower the background of false recombinants. The vectors also allow biochemical and biological selection. Transmission of the inserts to plasmid and single-stranded forms is performed by a simple procedure. The use of partial filling in of free cleavage ends following circularization (Fig. 2B) confers two advantages: it eliminates the use of the *sup*F marker with its drawbacks, and ligation of noncircular products to the vector arms are prevented. In addition, we use *Not*I digestion for cloning of the jumping inserts; thus the majority of DNA molecules do not participate in the ligation reaction with vector arms but remain as circular molecules. As a consequence of these modifications only 1–2 μg of vector arms need be packaged to obtain a representative jumping library.

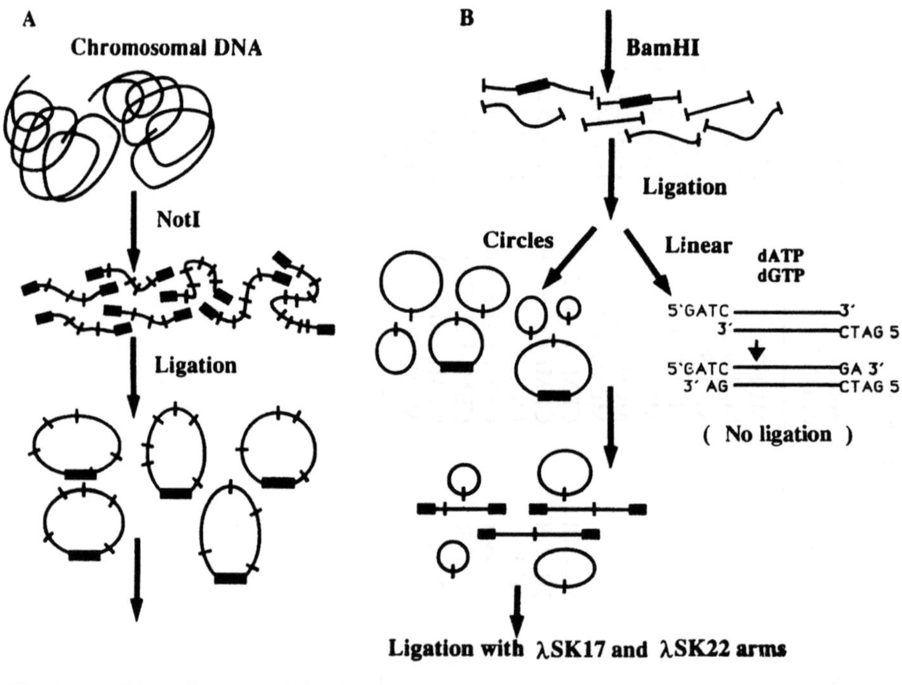

Fig. 2A, B. Flow diagram of the cloning procedure. *Black bars*, *Not*I sites; *vertical slashes*, *Bam*HI sites. **A, B** Construction of the jumping library. **B** Construction of the linking library. In this case digestion of the genomic DNA with *Bam*HI is the first step

CpG Islands

Although human DNA is highly methylated, stably unmethylated sequences (about 1% of the genome) have been observed in human chromosomal DNA [1]. Such sequences occur as discrete "islands," usually 1–2 kbp long, that are dispersed in the genome. Their distinctive feature is the presence of non-methylated CpG sequences at high density; this is the reason why they are usually called CpG-rich islands. No extensive sequence homologies have been observed among the approximately 30 000 different CpG-rich islands, having an average spacing about one per 100 kbp. It is now clear that many (if not all) CpG islands are associated with genes, and particularly with the 5′ ends of them. Our preliminary results also suggest that a majority of the *Not*I linking clones do contain conserved sequences as they have homologous sequences in the mouse genome, and many of them are expressed in humans. Two of three randomly selected *Not*I linking clones checked expressed in human placenta and in the human fibroblast cell line WI-38. One of them has been localized in the 3p21–p22 region. This clone has cell cycle dependent expression as determined in synchronized WI-38 cell line. Highly elevated expression was observed in the G_0 stage of the cell cycle (in contact inhibition or during growth arrest by depletion of serum from culture medium). These results also support the appropriateness of our approach to isolate functional genes by cloning CpG islands. A physical map for chromosome 3 using the new strategy is under construction based on our development in the technology of creating jumping/linking libraries and the deduction that CpG islands should be used as landmarks for mapping (Fig. 1). The strategy is based on the following points. (a) Restriction maps are constructed via conventional hybridization techniques of DNA separated by pulsed field gel electrophoresis with *Not*I jumping/linking clones isolated from defined regions of chromosome 3. (b) Tagging sequences adjacent to *Not*I sites in randomly sequenced linking and jumping clones are determined. Subsequently the linear order of the *Not*I sites on chromosome 3 will be established by sequencing approximately 1000 clones from each jumping and linking libraries and aligning them by using a computer program. (c) Contigs also on YAC clones will be established by the application of the linking/jumping clones.

Cloning of Gene Segments Corresponding to the Deleted Region of the Chromosome Using Alu Polymerase Chain Reaction and Subtractive Procedures

Alu polymerase chain reaction (PCR) has been used successfully to achieve molecular probes from defined regions of the genome [10]. This approach permits cloning small DNA fragments (500 bp) between Alu sequences. Alu sequences are distributed in a random fashion and are not linked with other markers. The Alu PCR is used in our approach not simply to generate genomic

DNA pieces from different sources but to amplify cloned fragments from our CpG-rich libraries. This modification has at least two advantages: (a) using the isolated PCR-amplified fragments as probes, it is easy to clone the parental linking clone (e.g., *Not*I) that is the natural marker on the chromosome convenient for linkage with other such markers, and (b) CpG-rich islands are usually located near or at the 5′ ends of the functioning genes.

Two experiments have been done in this direction. In one we used cloned DNA isolated from library no. 1 (complete chromosome 3) and library no. 7 (constructed from microcell hybrid line carrying chromosome 3 del 3p13–p22 in lambda form). In the second we used total DNA isolated from plasmid grid no. 1 (complete chromosome 3) and grid no. 2 (chromosome 3, del 3p13–p22). In both cases different Alu-specfic primers in different combinations were used for PCR reaction. Products of the PCR reactions were loaded on the low melting point agarose gel and run in such manner that products specific for whole chromosome 3 were adjacent to the products specific for chromosome 3 del 3p13–p22 using similar conditions. In such case it is not difficult to identify bands present in one sample (whole chromosome 3) and absent in another (chromosome 3 del 3p13–p22). Bands absent from del 3p14–p22 were isolated, labeled, and used for screening of the grids containing *Not*I linking clones specific for whole chromosome 3 (no. 1 and grid with lambda phages). In the first experiment 55 *Not*I linking clones were isolated. These clones were divided into eight groups. Checking representatives from each group showed that only clones from one of the groups were located outside the deleted region. This clone has been isolated due to a polymorphic *Bam*HI site in this region. In the second experiment 27 plasmid clones were isolated. They were divided into six groups. All of them were present in grid no. 1 and absent in grid no. 2. We have also developed method combining Alu PCR and differential screening. Using this approach, many *Not*I linking clones can be mapped to the defined regions of the chromosome simultaneously. We have tested this approach using grids no. 1 and no. 2. All clones checked so far (nine) originated in the deleted region.

Although subtractive methods represent potentially powerful tools for identification of deleted sequences, including tumor suppressor genes, they have not been applied extensively to tumor suppressor gene isolation, probably due to the great complexity of the human genome. This approach has provided rewarding results in less complex species such as yeast and *E. coli*. The complexity of the *Not*I linking library is at least 100 times lower than the complexity of the whole human genome. It is approximately equal in complexity to the yeast genome. We suggest using the same methodology (the use of linking libraries instead of genomic DNA) for genomic subtraction. Since this approach is not linked with Alu repeats, it allows the isolation of *Not*I linking clones, which are unavailable for cloning using Alu PCR. We expect that this new approach, due to the decreased complexity of the system, will open a practical possibility to clone-deleted sequences. We are now testing various modifications to find the most optimal procedure but can already show that in at least one modification it is working. Total DNA was isolated from *Not*I linking libraries no. 1 (contains complete chromosome 3) and no. 7 (contains chromosome 3 with deletion in region 3p13–p22). Each DNA was digested with *Sau*3A and ligated with linkers. These DNAs, in the presence of total human DNA, were hybridized separately to nylon filters containing immobilized human DNA. Under such conditions vector and mouse and human repetitive DNAs are not able to hybridize to DNA bound to the nylon filters. The hybridizing DNA sequences were amplified using PCR and used as a probe for hybridization with plasmid grid no. 1. Up to now we have checked ten clones that hybridize differently to these two probes. For eight of them we have already proven that they are from the deleted region; two other probes hybridize to the same bands in human and mouse DNA and need further investigation. The results clearly demonstrate the feasibility of Alu PCR and genomic subtraction for isolating CpG islands from defined regions of the genome.

A Shot-Gun Sequencing Strategy for Long-Range Genome Mapping

The main points of the approach are the following. (a) Essentially the same scheme is employed to construct *Not*I linking and jumping libraries. These two types of libraries contain the same DNA fragments but are differently arranged. (b) The *Not*I sites are adjacent to the direct and reverse sequencing primers in the vector arms of both types of libraries. By performing simple sequencing reactions, information about 500–600 bp surrounding each *Not*I site can easily be obtained without any recloning procedure.

The human chromosome 3 contains 200–300 *Not*I sites. Random sequencing of 600–1000 clones from each (linking and jumping) library will give STS information about a considerable fraction of all these *Not*I sites. Subsequently the linear order of the *Not*I clones on chromosome 3 can be established using a computer program. The same approach can be used to construct a *Not*I map for the entire human genome. The fact that isolation of chromosome-specific clones by hybridization is not needed simplifies the process. The occurrence of numerous repeats in the human genome is not expected to create excessive difficulties since the sequence data provides a tool to discriminate between different representatives of the same class of repeats.

After completing the *Not*I restriction map, a more detailed map (100–300 kbp resolution) can be constructed using *Xma*III, the recognition site of which is nested within the *Not*I site. Other enzymes (*Sal*I, *Xho*I) can also be used to create linking/jumping libraries with these vectors. More than 500 clones have been already sequenced. Altogether (for unique clones only) we have sequenced more than 160 000 bp. Fourteen discovered contigs covered 60 *Not*I fragments (20%–25% of the chromosome 3). STS for 150 unique *Not*I sites have been established, 220 *Not*I linking clones have been mapped (Fig. 3). We have started to analyze information obtained using a computer program developed

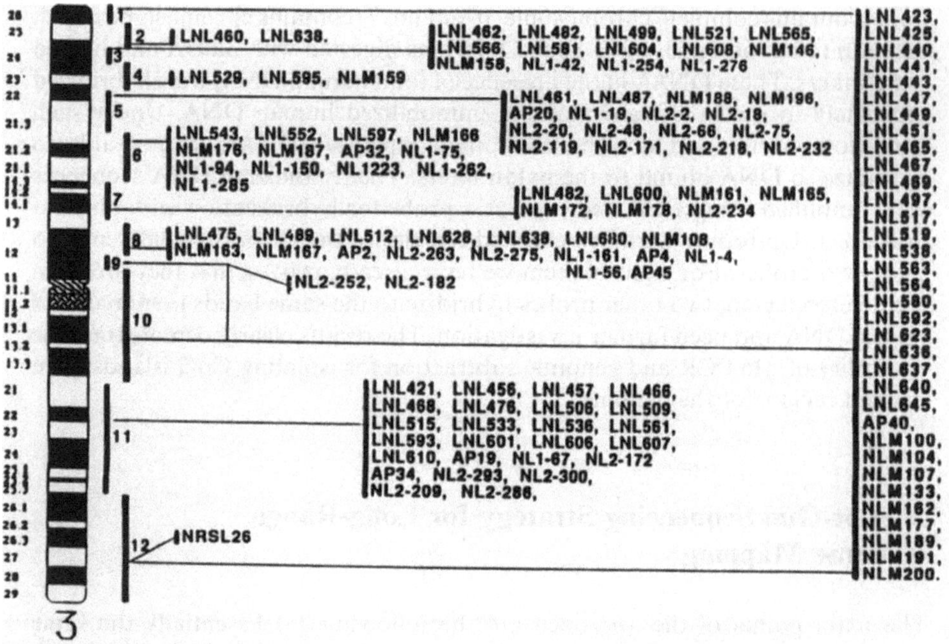

Fig.3. Localization of the 134 *Not*I linking clones on the human chromosome 3

by us. Preliminary analysis shows that all *Not*I linking clones contain SP1 binding sites (RNA polymerase II transcription factor), and that six of them contain p53 binding sites.

Acknowledgements. This investigation was supported by the Swedish Cancer Society, by PHS grant no. 5 RO1 CA14054-15, awarded by the National Cancer Institute, DHHS, and by grants from the Cancer Research Institute/Concern Foundation for Cancer Research, Concern II Foundation, Russian National Human Genome Programme and Russian-Swedish Research Cooperation between Russian Academy of Science and the Royal Swedish Academy of Science. I.K. was supported by Swedish Institute and E.S.P. by the Wenner Gren Foundation; G.W. acknowledges the support of a UICC/ACS Cancer Research Fellowship and is the recipient of a grant from the Magnus Bergwall Foundation, Stockholm, Sweden.

References

1. Bird AP (1987) CpG islands as gene markers in the vertebrate nucleus. Trends Genet 3: 342–347
2. Collins FS (1988) Chromosome jumping. In: Davis KE (ed) Genome analysis: a practical approach. IRL Press, Oxford, pp 73–94
3. Devilee P, van den Broek M, Kuipers-Dijksnoorn N, Kolluri R, Meera Khan P, Pearson PL, Cornelisse CJ (1989) At least four different chromosomal regions are involved in loss of heterozygosity in human breast carcinoma. Genomics 5: 554–560

4. Ernberg I, Falk K, Minarovits J, Busson P, Tursz T, Masucci MG, Klein G (1989) The role of methylation in the phenotype-dependent modulation of Epstein-Barr nuclear antigen 2 and latent membrane protein genes in cells latently infected with Epstein-Barr virus. J Gen Virol 70: 2989–3002
5. Ito T, Sakaki Y (1988) A novel procedure for selective cloning of *Not*I linking fragments from mammalian genomes. Nucleic Acids Res 16: 9177–9184
6. Kovacs G, Erlandsson R, Boldog F, Ingvarsson S, Muller-Brechlin R, Klein G, Sumegi J (1988) Consistent chromosome 3p deletion and loss of heterozygosity in renal cell carcinoma. Proc Natl Acad Sci USA 85: 1571–1575
7. Kovacs G, Frisch S (1989) Clonal chromosome abnormalities in tumor cells from patients with sporadic renal cell carcinomas. Cancer Res 49: 651–659
8. Morton NE (1991) Parameters of the human genome. Proc Natl Acad Sci USA 88: 7474–7476
9. Naylor SL, Johnson BE, Minna JD, Sakaguchi AY (1987) Loss of heterozygosity of chromosome 3p markers in small-cell lung cancer. Nature 329: 451–454
10. Nelson DL, Ledbetter SA, Corbo L, Victoria MF, Ramirez-Solis R, Webster TD, Ledbetter DH, Caskey CT (1989) A method for rapid isolation of human-specific sequences from complex DNA sources. Proc Natl Acad Sci USA 86: 6686–6690
11. Pohl TM, Zimmer M, MacDonald ME, Smith B, Bucan M, Poustka A, Volinia S, Searle S, Zehetner G, Wasmuth JJ, Gusells J, Lehrach H, Frischauf A-M (1988) Construction of a *Not*I linking library and isolation of new markers close to the Huntington's disease gene. Nucleic Acids Res 19: 9185–9198
12. Poustka A, Lehrach H (1988) Chromosome jumping: a long range cloning technique. In: Setlow JK (ed) Genetic engineering principles and methods, vol 10. Brookhaven National laboratory, Plenum, New York, pp 169–193
13. Seizinger BR et al. (1988) Von Hippel-Lindau disease maps to the region of chromosome 3 associated with renal cell carcinoma. Nature 332: 268–269
14. Wallace MR, Fountain JW, Brereton AM, Collins FS (1989) Direct construction of a chromosome-specific *Not*I linking library from flow-sorted chromosomes. Nucleic Acids Res 17: 1665–1671
15. Zabarovsky ER, Boldog F, Thompson T, Scanlon D, Winberg G, Marcsek Z, Erlandsson R, Stanbridge EJ, Klein G, Sumegi J (1990) Construction of a human chromosome 3 specific Not I linking library using a novel cloning procedure. Nucleic Acids Res 18: 6319–6324
16. Zabarovsky ER, Winberg G, Boldog F, Turina OV, Nurbekov MK, Marcsek Z, Erlandsson R, Grigorieva A, Stanbridge EJ, Sümegi J, Kisselev LL, Klein G (1991) New generation of vectors for cloning and mapping of the human genome. Adv Mol Gen 4: 281–293
17. Zabarovsky ER, Boldog F, Erlandsson R, Kashuba VI, Allikmets RL, Marcsek Z, Stanbridge E, Sümegi G, Klein G, Winberg G (1991) A new strategy for mapping the human genome based on a novel procedure for constructing jumping libraries. Genomics 11: 1030–1039

Molecular Analysis of Different Loci on Chromosomes 3, 5, and 17 in Sporadic Renal Cell Carcinoma

H. BRAUCH[1], T. SCHADT[2], T. HIERONYMUS[2], D. KOMITOWSKI[1], and S. POMER[2]

Introduction

The short arm of chromosome 3 (3p) is the prime target for genetic changes in renal cell carcinoma (RCC). There is growing evidence that different tumor suppressor genes on 3p account for the different forms of RCC, hereditary and sporadic. The hallmark of sporadic RCC is loss of 3p sequences in the DNA of tumors. Loss at 3p was detected in over 90% of the tumors studied both by analyses of human tumor karyotypes [11] and by molecular analyses of DNA isolated from sporadic RCC [20]. Several hereditary forms of RCC are characterized by chromosome 3 involvement. RCC develops in members of families who inherit a chromosomal translocation from one parent. The translocation always involves chromosome 3. Families with translocations t(3;8) [4], t(3;11) [15], and t(3;6) [12] have been described. Individuals in these families who inherit a translocation chromosome develop RCC. The breakpoints of the reported translocations cluster around 3p14.

Von Hippel-Lindau (VHL) disease is another hereditary condition in which RCC is part of a syndrome. In the course of this disease affected individuals may develop retinal angioma, cerebellar and spinal hemangioblastoma, pheochromocytoma, tumor of the epidydemis, and RCC. The gene involved in this disease is genetically linked to the region 3p25–26 [6, 17]. Molecular analyses of VHL tumors allow assessment of the haplotype of the deleted wild type and the retained mutated 3p allele and have led to the general acceptance that the VHL gene is a tumor suppressor gene [18]. There is no clear evidence of whether the same tumor suppressor gene involved in VHL is also involved in the development of sporadic RCC.

[1] Institut für Pathologie der Technischen Universität, Labor für Molekulare Pathologie, Trogerstr. 32, D-81675 München, Germany
[2] Chirurgische Universitätsklinik, Abteilung Urologie, Im Neuenheimer Feld 110, D-69120 Heidelberg, Germany

Tumor Suppressor Genes

Today's view of tumorigenesis is based on two models: The two mutation theory of carcinogenesis [10] and the multistep development of tumorigenesis [5]. According to these models, tumor suppressor genes play a crucial role in normal development and differentiation. Each normal cell contains a set of homologous alleles, one of paternal and one of maternal origin. Knudson [10] has suggested a recessive mode of action for the inactivation of the two copies of a tumor suppressor gene. Loss of function of a tumor suppressor gene follows after a mutation in the gene or the physical loss of the gene. Two mutations must occur sequentially in order to inactivate the two homologous genes. Whether a disease is hereditary or sporadic depends on the acquisition of these homologous mutations. In hereditary diseases the first mutation is present in the germline cells and can be passed from a parent to offspring. This germline mutation is followed by a somatic mutation, inactivating the second tumor suppressor allele and consequently releasing the cell from its normal phenotype onto the tumorigenic pathway. In sporadic diseases both homologous mutations must be acquired somatically. Thus the cell changes from a normal to a tumorigenic phenotype.

In the course of tumorigenesis several genetic changes may corroborate, marking the development and the progression of cancer. Vogelstein has suggested a model for the development of colorectal carcinoma that explains the different phenotypic changes by accumulating genetic changes. Transformation of normal epithelium to benign hyperplasia and of adenomas to malignant carcinoma and invasive metastasis progresses following a mutation in the Ki-*ras* oncogene and changes that affect tumor suppressor genes on chromosomes 5, 18, and 17. Identification of the different tumor suppressor genes and their mutations involved in colorectal carcinoma have supported and multistep concept of tumorigenesis and have encouraged researchers to extend this model to other neoplasms to explain their development and progression.

To determine the involvement and potential role of tumor suppressor genes in the development of sporadic RCC we selected three different chromosomal locations for molecular analyses that are known to contain tumor suppressor genes. The short arm of chromosome 3 carries the VHL gene [6, 17]. The long arm of chromosome 5 contains the gene mutated in colorectal carcinoma (MCC) [8] and the gene mutated in patients with familial adenomatous polyposis coli (FAP) [9]. The short arm of chromosome 17 holds the p53 gene which is mutated in many different tumors [13]. We analyzed pairs of normal and tumor DNA from 28 patients with sporadic RCC for loss of heterozygosity (LOH) by restriction fragment length polymorphism (RFLP) analysis, as described previously [2].

Loss of Heterozygosity on the Short Arm of Chromosome 3

We compared normal DNA with tumor DNA at six loci on 3p (Table 1). The loci were D3S4 (B67), D3S2 (pHF12-32), D3S32 (pYNZ145.1), D3F15S2 (pH2H3), *THRB* (3p24) [7], and D3S18 (c-LIB-1) [6]. Of 27 evaluable RCCs 26

Table 1. Loss of heterozygosity on the short arm of chromosome 3 in sporadic RCC

Probe	Symbol	Location	*n*	Het	LOH	
					n	%
B67	D3S4	3pter–q21	15	5	1	20
pHF12-32	D3S2	3p21	25	10	9	90
pEFD145.1	D3S32	3p	24	12	12	100
pH3H2	D3F15S2	3p21	25	12	11	91
pBH302	*THRB*	3p24.1–32	24	13	10	71
CRI-L162[a] c-LIB-1[a]	D3S18	3p26	24	15	14	93
Total			28	27	26	96

Het, number of patients heterozygous; LOH, number of patients with loss of heterozygosity.
[a] DNA probes that link to the VHL gene.

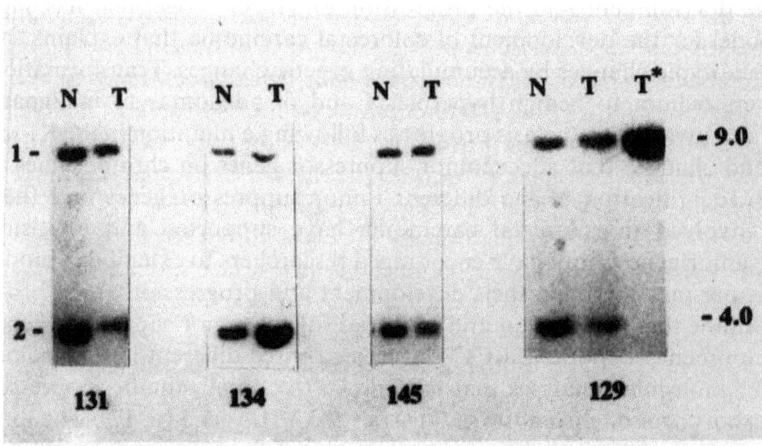

Fig. 1. Loss of heterozygosity at the D3S32 locus on the short arm of chromosome 3. Representative autoradiographs of Southern blot filters. DNA was isolated from tumor and normal tissue of patients with sporadic RCC. DNA was digested with *Taq*I, fractionated on agarose gel electrophoresis, and transferred to a nylon membrane. After hybridization with radiolabeled pEFD 145.1 the probe detected two polymorphic bands at 9.0 and 4.0 kb. For each patient normal and tumor DNA was compared. The normal DNA (*N*) of patients 131, 134, 145, and 129 was heterozygous. The tumor DNA (*T*) lost one of the two polymorphic alleles. LOH shows as a reduction in signal intensity. The in vitro culture of tumor (*T**) of patient 129 had complete loss of allele 2, suggesting that the residual signal in the primary tumor was due to contamination by normal cells

(96%) showed LOH at one or more 3p loci. We found LOH at the proximal locus D3S4 at a frequency of 20%. All other loci showed higher frequencies (71%–100%), suggesting that the tumor DNA loses an extensive part of one 3p allele. Our observation of 96% LOH at 3p in DNA from sporadic RCCs is in agreement with results reported earlier [1, 20].

Figure 1 illustrates LOH at locus D3S32 (3p21). The normal DNA of all patients was informative, that is, heterozygous for allele 1 (9.0 kb) and allele 2 (4.0 kb). The tumor DNA (T) of patients 131, 134, 145, and 129 showed reduction in signal intensities at one allele, suggesting LOH. Complete loss of allele 2 was demonstrated in the DNA of an in vitro culture of tumor 129 (T*), suggesting that the tumor cells had lost this allele. The residual signal in the primary tumor resulted from a contamination by normal cells.

Figure 2 gives similar results obtained at the D3S18 locus (3p26). D3S18 is one of the flanking loci for the VHL disease. All patients were heterozygous for allele 1 (8.4 kb) and allele 2 (4.7 kb). Patient 26 had a complete loss of allele 1 in

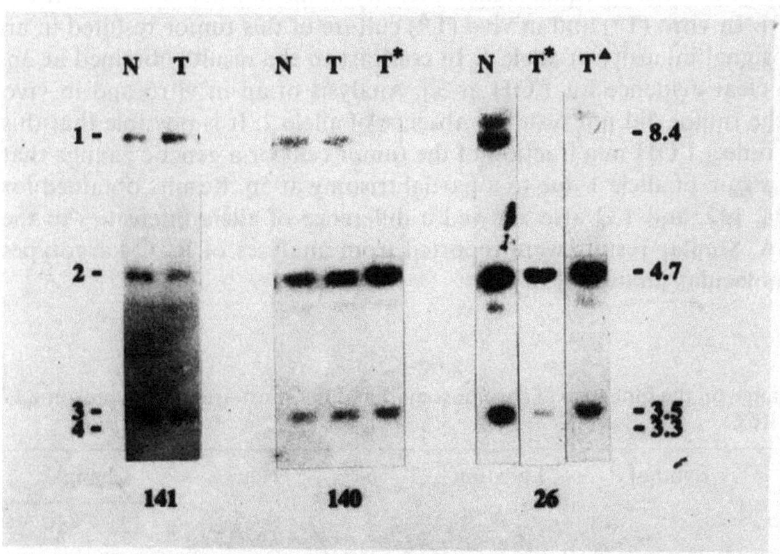

Fig. 2. Loss of heterozygosity at the D3S18 locus on the short arm of chromosome 3. Autoradiographs of Southern blot filters. DNA was isolated from normal tissue, primary tumor, in vitro culture and in vivo culture of tumors of patients with sporadic RCC. DNA was digested with *Bam*HI, fractionated on agarose gel electrophoresis, and transferred to a nylon membrane. After hybridization to radiolabeled probe c-LIB-1 the probe detected two polymorphic systems. Alleles 1 and 2 at 8.4 and 4.7 kb and alleles 3 and 4 at 3.5 and 3.3 kb. The normal DNA (*N*) of patients 141, 140, and 26 was heterozygous for allele 1 and 2. The tumor DNA (*T*) of patient 141 had a reduced signal intensity at allele 2. The tumor DNA (*T*) of patient 140 had reduced signal intensity at allele 1. The in vitro (*T**) culture of this tumor showed complete absence of allele 1, suggesting that the residual signal in the primary tumor was due to contamination by normal cells. Both the in vitro (*T**) and in vivo (*T*▲) culture of the RCC of patient 26 had complete loss of allele 1.All patients were homozygous for allele 3

the in vitro (T*) and in vivo (T▲) culture of this tumor. A reduction in signal intensity at allele 1 in the primary tumor of patient 140 was observed. The same allele was completely absent in the in vitro culture (T*), suggesting that the tumor cells had lost this 3p allele. Patient 141 had a reduced signal at allele 2 in the primary tumor. No purified tumor cells were available.

Molecular Changes on the Long Arm of Chromosome 5

RFLP analysis was carried out at four loci on the long arm of chromosome 5 (Table 2). The loci tested were D5S81 (cYN5.48), D5S141 (cL5.71), D5S36 (JO157E-A), and D5S43 (lambda MS8) [7]. The probe cL5.71 is a genomic clone of the MCC gene, and both cL5.71 and cYN5.48 are genetically linked to the gene for FAP [9]. Changes were observed at all four loci. Of 26 evaluable patients 14 (53%) had changes in their tumor DNA. Figure 3 illustrates differences in allele intensities at three loci at 5q in patients 26, 134, 142, and 132. Patient 26 had 2 alleles of equal signal intensity in his normal DNA (N) at the locus D5S81. In vitro (T*) and in vivo (T▲) culture of this tumor resulted in an increase of signal intensity at allele 1. In contrast to the results obtained at 3p, there is no clear evidence for LOH at 5q. Analysis of an in vitro and in vivo culture of the tumor did not result in absence of allele 2. It is possible that this may either reflect LOH in a fraction of the tumor cells or a genetic change that resulted in a gain of allele 1 due to a partial trisomy at 5q. Results obtained for patients 134, 142, and 132 also showed a difference of allele intensities in the tumor DNA. Similar results were reported from analyses of RCC karyotypes [11] and molecular analyses [14].

Table 2. Change on the long arm of chromosome 5 and the short arm of chromosome 17 in sporadic RCC

Probe	Symbol	Location	*n*	Het	Change	
					n	%
cYN5.48[a]	D5S81	5q21	23	10	4	40
cL5.71-3[a,b]	D5S141	5q21	24	10	2	20
JO157E-A	D5S36	5q32-qter	26	14	4	28.5
Lambda MS8	D5S43	5q35-qter	25	20	10	50
Total			28	26	14	53
pYNZ22.1	D17S5	17p13.3	19	17	6	35

Het, number of patients heterozygous; change, number of patients with a difference in signal intensity or loss of heterozygosity.
[a] DNA probes link to FAP gene.
[b] Genomic clone of MCC gene.

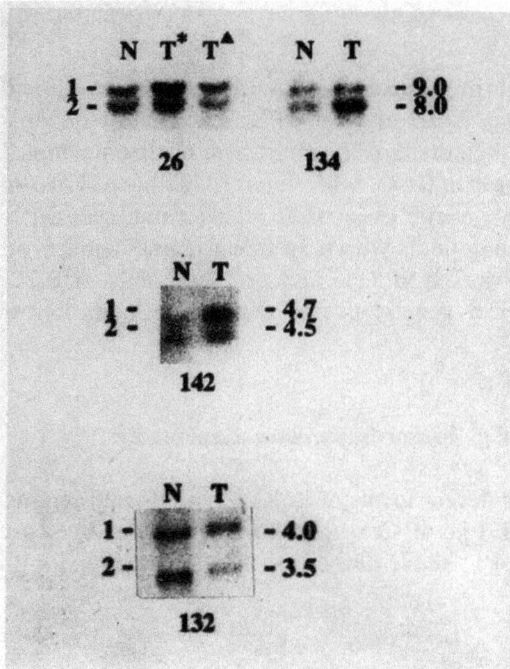

Fig. 3. RFLP analysis on chromosome 5q in sporadic RCC at loci D5S81, D5S141, and D5S36. Autoradiographs of Southern blot filters. DNA was isolated from tumors and normal tissue, digested with *Msp*I, fractionated on agarose gel electrophoresis, and transferred to a nylon membrane. The filter was hybridized consecutively to three radiolabeled probes. The probe cYN5.48 detects alleles of 9.0 and 8.0 kb at D5S81; cL5.71 detects alleles of 4.7 and 4.5 kb at D5S141; JO157E-A detects alleles of 4.0 and 3.5 at D5S36. For each patient normal and tumor DNA was compared. The normal DNA (*N*) of patient 26 and 134 was heterozygous at locus D5S81. Tumor DNA (*T*) of patient 134 showed an increase in signal intensity at allele 2. DNA of the in vitro (*T**) and in vivo (*T*▲) culture of the tumor of patient 26 showed an increase in signal intensity at allele 1. Selection of tumor cells in culture did not result in loss of one allele, indicating that the increase in signal intensity may rather reflect a partial trisomy and not LOH. Similar results were obtained for patient 142 at locus D5S141 and for patient 132 at locus D5S36

Molecular Changes on the Short Arm of Chromosome 17

RFLP analysis was carried out at D17S5 (17p13.3). The probe pYNZ22.1 detects a polymorphism consisting of various numbers of tandem repeats [7]. Of 19 patients 17 were evaluable. The primary tumor of six patients (35%) had a reduction in signal intensity at one allele (not shown). The in vitro culture of tumor 129 showed complete absence of allele 1, suggesting that the molecular change involved on chromosome 17 is due to LOH (not shown). We found this change in 35% of the evaluable patients, compared to 9% reported in the literature [1].

Conclusion

We found molecular changes on all three chromosomal regions that we studied which carry tumor suppressor genes. LOH at 3p in 96% of evaluable patients confirmed previous results, which suggests that the short arm of chromosome 3 is the prime target for genetic changes in RCC. Since most RCCs have LOH on 3p, this change may be a primary genetic event that affects renal cells early during tumorigenesis. Not all of the patients with a 3p deletion had changes on 5q and 17p. Changes at 5q were observed in 53% and on 17p in 35% of RCC. These changes may therefore reflect genetic events that occur later in the tumorigenic pathway.

Location of a Putative Sporadic RCC Tumor Suppressor Gene on 3p

Genetic events so far identified in different forms of RCC affect different regions on the short arm of chromosome 3 (Fig. 4). Chromosomal regions involved are 3p25–26 in VHL disease and 3p14 in those hereditary RCCs associated with

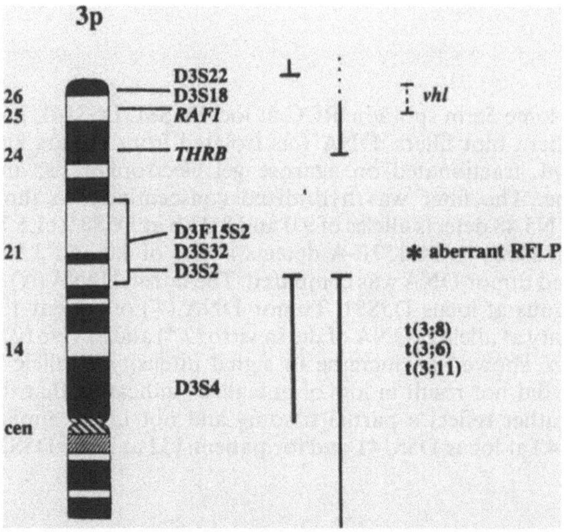

Fig. 4. Aberrant RFLP pattern in the normal DNA of a patient with sporadic RCC at locus D3S32. The probe pEFD145.1 detects a *Taq*I polymorphism at D3S32 of 9.0 and 4.0 kb. The constitutional DNA of normal individuals is either homozygous for allele 1 (*lane 1*) or allele 2 (*lane 3*) or heterozygous for both alleles (*lane 2*). The RFLP pattern obtained from normal kidney of patient 159 differed from that of the three normal patterns. The two fragments migrated at a distance of allele 1 (9.0 kb) and of 8.0 kb. The 8.0-kb fragment may be due to a mutation in one of the homologous wild-type alleles in the precursor cells of the RCC. A mutation may have affected either allele 1, if the patient was originally homozygous for this allele, or allele 2, if the patient was heterozygous. The tumor DNA showed a reduction in signal intensity of the wild-type allele 1, suggesting loss of allele 1 in the tumor and retention of the mutated allele

chromosome 3 translocations. These regions are located at opposite ends outside of the commonly deleted region in sporadic RCC. Based on two deletion maps reported in the literature, this commonly deleted area spans the region between D3S2 and *THRB* [1, 19]. This region accounts for approximately 40% of the total length of 3p, thus presenting a difficulty to identification of the RCC gene. In order to apply modern molecular techniques such as chromosome walking or jumping this region should be further narrowed. Since the number of tumors is limited, and the tumors have rather large deletions, it is important to search for additional possibilities that allow the approach of a specific gene of interest. There are examples in which abnormal hybridization patterns at chromosomal regions of interest have been useful in that attempt. In the case of sporadic colon carcinoma a rearrangement in the commonly deleted area at 5q provides an aberrant sequence, cloning of which has lead to identification of the MCC gene [8]. In small-cell lung carcinoma (SCLC) extensive 3p deletions have been found, but a SCLC gene has not yet been identified [3]. Recently a homozygous deletion was identified in a SCLC cell line at the D3S3 locus [16]. This homozygous deletion is located within the commonly deleted area in SCLC and may point to a specific location involved in the development of SCLC. It would be desirable to identify such aberrant hybridization patterns in sporadic RCC that could aid identification of the RCC gene.

We found an abnormal RFLP pattern in the normal DNA of a patient with sporadic RCC at the D3S32 locus (Fig. 5). Normal RFLP alleles migrate at a

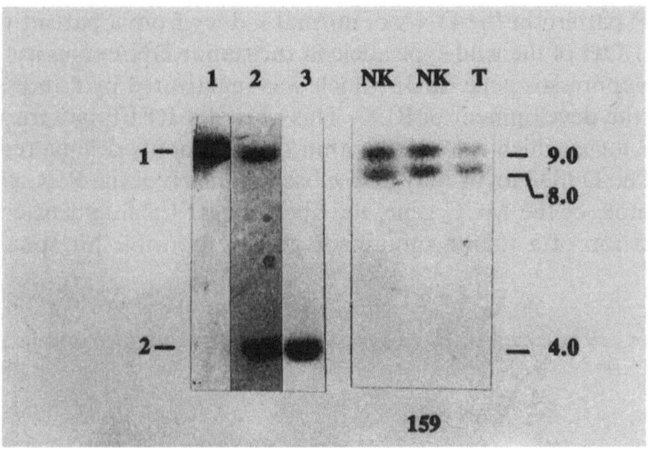

Fig. 5. Genetic events in RCC on the short arm of chromosome 3. *Vertical bars*, two deletion maps on the short arm of chromosome 3 obtained in sporadic RCC [1, 19]. The commonly deleted area extends between loci D3S2 and *THRB*. Regions affected in hereditary RCC are at 3p14 in patients with translocations t(3;8) [4], t(3;6) [12], and t(3;11) [15] and 3p25–26 in patients with VHL disease [6, 17]. Both 3p regions involved in hereditary RCC are located outside the commonly deleted region in sporadic RCC. An aberrant RFLP pattern was identified in a patient with sporadic RCC at locus D3S32. This locus is located within the region commonly deleted in sporadic RCC

distance of 9.0 and 4.0 kb. Individuals may be homozygous either for allele 1 or allele 2, or heterozygous for both alleles. Patient 159 had two bands in his normal DNA. One fragment matched the size of the normal allele 1; the other migrated at a distance of 8.0 kb and did not match any of the normal alleles. This aberrant RFLP pattern can be explained by a mutation that affected one of the two wild-type alleles in the precursor cells of this RCC. Since a normal cell contains two of each allele, there are two possibilities to explain this aberrant RFLP pattern. One possibility is that patient 159 originally was homozygous for allele 1, and that one of the identical alleles was subsequently mutated, resulting in a smaller fragment. The second possibility is that patient 159 was heterozygous for allele 1 and 2, but that allele 2 was mutated, resulting in a larger fragment. The resulting pattern of two bands of equal signal intensity in the DNA of the "normal" kidney allowed distinction of the two alleles in the tumor precursor cells. Analysis of the DNA isolated from the RCC of patient 159 revealed the same fragments found in the DNA isolated from the kidney. We observed a reduction in signal intensity of allele 1, the wild-type allele, and retention of allele 2, the mutated allele. This result suggests that LOH occurs at the wild-type allele, leaving both alleles of the putative tumor suppressor gene inactivated.

Conclusion

The aberrant RFLP pattern in the DNA of normal kidney from a patient with sporadic RCC and LOH of the wild-type allele in the tumor DNA supports the notion of a tumor suppressor gene on 3p which was inactivated by a recessive mechanism during the development of RCC. This aberrant RFLP pattern was found at the D3S32 locus which is located within the commonly deleted region in sporadic RCC. The D3S32 locus may be a close landmark of the RCC gene. Following the example of the MCC gene, the aberrant RFLP fragment could aid in the identification of a tumor suppressor gene responsible for spoardic RCC.

Acknowledgement. We are indebted to H. Löhrke for establishing in vitro and in vitro cultures of RCCs.

References

1. Anglard P, Tory K, Brauch H et al. (1991) Molecular analysis of genetic changes in the origin and development of renal cell carcinoma. Cancer Res 51: 1071–1077
2. Brauch H, Tory K, Hosoe S et al. (1992) Molecular analysis of DNA sequences on chromosome 3 in patients with renal cell carcinoma. In: Staehler G, Pomer S (eds) Basic and clinical research on renal cell carcinoma. Springer, Berlin Heidelberg New York

3. Brauch H, Tory K, Kotler F (1990) Molecular mapping of deletion sites in the short arm of chromosome 3 in human lung cancer. Genes Chrom Cancer 1: 240–246
4. Cohen AJ, Li FP, Berg S et al. (1979) Hereditary renal cell carcinoma associated with a chromosomal translocation. N Engl J Med 301: 592–595
5. Fearon ER, Vogelstein B (1990) A genetic model for colorectal tumorigenesis. Cell 61: 759–767
6. Hosoe S, Brauch H, Latif F et al. (1990) Localization of the von Hippel-Lindau disease gene to a small region of chromosome 3. Genomics 8: 634–640
7. Human Gene Mapping 10 (1989) Cytogenetics and cell genetics 51: 671, 675, 693, 695, 792
8. Kinzler KW, Nilbert MC, Vogelstein B (1990) Identification of a gene located at chromosome 5q21 that is mutated in colorectal cancers. Science 251: 1366–1370
9. Kinzler KW, Nilbert MC, Su LK et al. (1991) Identification of FAP locus genes from chromosome 5q21. Science 253: 661–664
10. Knudson AG Jr (1972) Mutation and cancer: a model for Wilms' tumor of the kidney. J Natl Cancer Inst 48: 313–324
11. Kovacs G, Szücs S, De Riese W, Baumgärtl H (1987) Specific chromosome aberration in human renal cell carcinoma. Int J Cancer 40: 171–178
12. Kovacs G (1990) Application of molecular cytogenetic technique to the evaluation of renal parenchymal tumors. J Cancer Res Clin Oncol 116: 318–323
13. Levine AJ, Momand J, Finlay CA (1992) The p53 tumor suppressor gene. Nature 351: 453–456
14. Morita R, Saito S, Ishikawa J et al. (1991) Common regions of deletion on chromosome 5q, 6q and 10q in renal cell carcinoma. Cancer Res 51: 5817–5820
15. Pathak S, Strong LC, Ferrell RE et al. (1982) Familial renal cell carcinoma with a 3;11 chromosome translocation limited to tumor cells. Science 217: 939–941
16. Rabbits P, Bergh J, Douglas J et al. (1990) A submicroscopic homozygous deletion at the D3S3 locus in a cell line isolated from a small cell lung carcinoma. Genes Chrom Cancer 2: 231–238
17. Seizinger BR, Rouleau GS, Ozelius LJ et al. (1988) Von Hippel-Lindau disease maps to the region of chromosome 3 associated with renal cell carcinoma. Nature 332: 268–269
18. Tory K, Brauch H, Linehan M et al. (1989) Specific genetic change in tumors associated with von Hippel-Lindau disease. J Natl Cancer Inst 81: 1097–1101
19. Van der Hout A, Van der Vlies P, Wijmenga C et al. (1991) The region of common allelic losses in sporadic renal cell carcinoma is bordered by the loci D3S2 and THRB. Genomics 11: 537–542
20. Zbar B, Brauch H, Talmadge C, Linehan M (1988) Loss of alleles of loci on the short arm of chromosome 3 in renal cell carcinoma. Nature 327: 721–724

Expression of Immediate Early Transcription Factors in Human Renal Cell Tumors

T. STROHMEYER[1,2], W. LEVIN[1], M. PRESS[3], P. EFFERT[4], and D. SLAMON[1]

Introduction

Initiation and progression of malignant growth is a multistep process. Various genes are likely to play potential roles in this process, of which cellular oncogenes and suppressor genes have recently been the focus of investigation. Cellular oncogenes are involved in the regulation of normal growth and/or differentiation and in the signal transduction pathway or in the transcriptional regulation of gene expression of diverse cellular genes. Transcription factors, representing proteins that regulate gene expression by binding to specific regulatory DNA sequences, have been implicated in oncogenesis since structural or functional changes in these factors may result in an altered expression of multiple genes, subsequently leading to changes in both growth properties and differentiation state of affected cells. The transcription factors c-*fos*, c-*jun*, and early response gene (*EGR-1*) are members of a class of proto-oncogenes known as immediate early genes. Genes belonging to this class are characterized by their mRNA levels being strongly induced by serum stimulation: within 20 min after serum stimulation of serum-starved 3T3 cells the mRNA levels of these genes are induced 40- to 50-fold. To date, little is known about the expression of these genes in primary human renal cell carcinomas [1].

The etiology of renal cell carcinomas is hardly understood, and the classical predictors of the patients outcome are unreliable in individual cases [2]. Thus, additional biological information is required and may be found on the molecular level. The current study was undertaken to detect alterations in the expression of transcript factors which may provide insights into initiation and/or progression of renal tumors and to evaluate any observed alterations for possible correlations with clinical parameters of the disease.

[1] Division of Hematology-Oncology, Department of Medicine and the Jonsson Comprehensive Cancer Center, U.C.L.A. School of Medicine, Los Angeles, CA 90024, USA
[2] Abteilung für Onkologie, Schering AG, D-13342 Berlin, Germany
[3] Department of Pathology, U.S.C. Medical Center, Los Angeles, CA 90033, USA
[4] Urologische Universitätsklinik, RWTH Aachen, Pauwelsstr. 30, D-52074 Aachen, Germany

Materials and Methods

Fresh renal tumor tissue and, whenever possible, adjacent non-malignant tissue from the renal cortex was obtained at the time of primary surgery and stored in liquid nitrogen or at $-70°C$. All specimens, tumor and normal, were examined histologically using hematoxylin/eosin staining. DNA and RNA was extracted from these specimens, purified, and quantitated by fluorometry prior to gel electrophoresis, as previously described [3].

Northern Blot Analysis. Total cellular RNA was extracted, quantitated, and processed as described [3]. The probes used in this study include; c-*fos*, 0.48-kb fragment; *EGR-1*, 2.2-kb *Eco*RI insert in pUC13; c-*jun*, 1.2-kb fragment. All c-DNA probes were ^{32}P-labeled using oligonucleotide random priming. Filters were subsequently stripped and rehybridized to a fragment of a human β-actin probe (603 bp *Baml*/*Eco*RI fragment) under identical hybridization and washing conditions. In addition, to ensure that equal amounts of RNA were loaded, the 18S and 28S ribosomal RNAs were compared as visualized by ethidium bromide staining.

Immunohistochemistry. Acetone-fixed, frozen sections of each specimen were stained with hematoxylin/eosin and examined microscopically to confirm the presence of tumor cells. Immunohistochemistry was performed on 5-μm acetone-fixed, frozen sections using c-*fos*, c-*jun*, and *EGR-1* rabbit polyclonal antisera and the peroxidase-antiperoxidase technique. The c-*fos* and c-*jun* antiserum was generated and characterized in our own laboratory; the *EGR-1* specific antiserum was generated from a bGM-EGR-1 fusion protein expressed in the plasmid V4, as previously described. Serial sections were treated with preimmune serum instead of immune serum as a negative control. All sections were counterstained with methylen blue to verify the presence of intact nuclei.

Results

DNA and RNA Extraction. Table 1 shows the grade and stage data of the renal cell tumors in this cohort. Sufficient quantities of RNA and DNA could be isolated from 47 tumors with adjacent nonmalignant renal tissues.

Pattern of Early Transcription Factor Expression. RNA from all 47 tumor/normal pairs was hybridized to the c-*fos*, c-*jun*, and *EGR-1* probes. The expression of the three genes in normal renal tissues was uniformly moderate in 37/47 (78%) of the examined specimens (Fig. 1). However, in four normal tissues no expression was detectable, and in six normal samples very high expression (more than five fold) was found. The early immediate genes were coregulated in 42/47 normal renal tissues (89%). Gene expression in the tumors was quantitated accordingly. A heterogeneous expression pattern was found in the tumor

Table 1. Tumor stages and grades of the renal cell carcinomas of this cohort

Stage	Grade (renal cell carcinomas)			
	I	II	III	Total
N0 M0	3	27	8	38
N1–3 M0	0	6	0	6
M1	0	3	0	3
Total	3	36	8	47

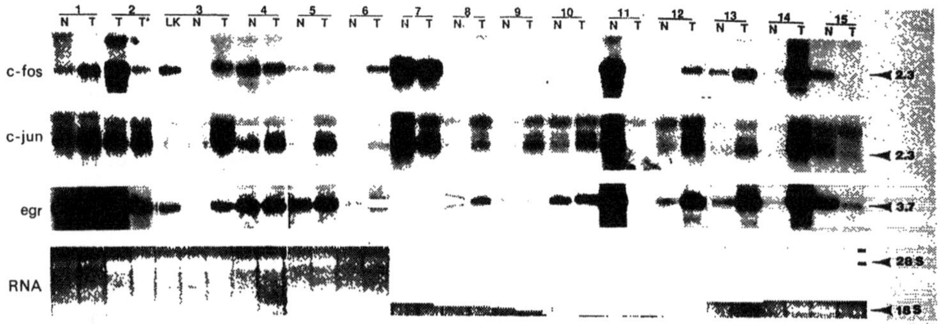

Fig. 1. Northern blot analysis demonstrating coordinate expression of c-*fos* (2.3-kb transcript), c-*jun* (2.3-kb transcript), and *EGR-1* (3.7-kb transcript). *T*, Renal tumor tissue; *T**, renal tumor of the contralateral kidney; *N*, corresponding normal renal tissue; *LK*, regional lymph node metastasis. c-*fos* expression in the tumor was higher in 17 (pairs 1, 3, 5, 6, 12–14), equal in 20 (pairs 4, 7–10), and lower in 10 (pairs 11, 15); c-*jun* expression in the tumor was higher in 22 (pairs 1, 3, 5, 6, 8–10, 12–14), equal in 16 (pair 4), and lower in 9 (pairs 7, 11, 15); *EGR-1* expression in the tumor was higher in 17 (pairs 1, 3, 6, 9, 12–14), equal in 17 (pairs 4, 5, 7, 8, 10), and lower in 13 (pairs 11, 15) – as compared to the corresponding normal tissues. The expression of the three genes was coordinate in most of the normal and malignant tissues, except in 1 N, 2 T*, 3 LK, pairs 8–10, 12 N, and 15 T

cohort; 50%–60% of the tumors had moderate, approximately 30% high, and approximately 10% no expression of the early immediate transcription factors on RNA level.

Relative gene expression in the tumors was scored as "higher," "equal," or "lower" with regards to levels found in the adjacent normal renal tissues (Table 2). Markedly higher mRNA levels of c-*fos*, c-*jun*, and *EGR-1* were demonstrated by northern analysis in almost 40% of the tumors when compared to their adjacent normal tissues. The early immediate genes were coregulated in 40/47 renal cell carcinomas (85%).

Immunohistochemistry. Protein expression was analyzed immunohistochemically using polyclonal antibodies. Eight pairs of malignant and normal renal

Table 2. Relative expression of the early immediate transcription factor mRNA in renal cell carcinomas as compared to the normal corresponding tissue of each tumor

Transcript factor	Relative mRNA expression: tumor/normal pairs			
	Higher	Equal	Lower	Total
c-*fos*	17	20	10	47
c-*jun*	22	16	9	47
EGR-1	17	17	13	47

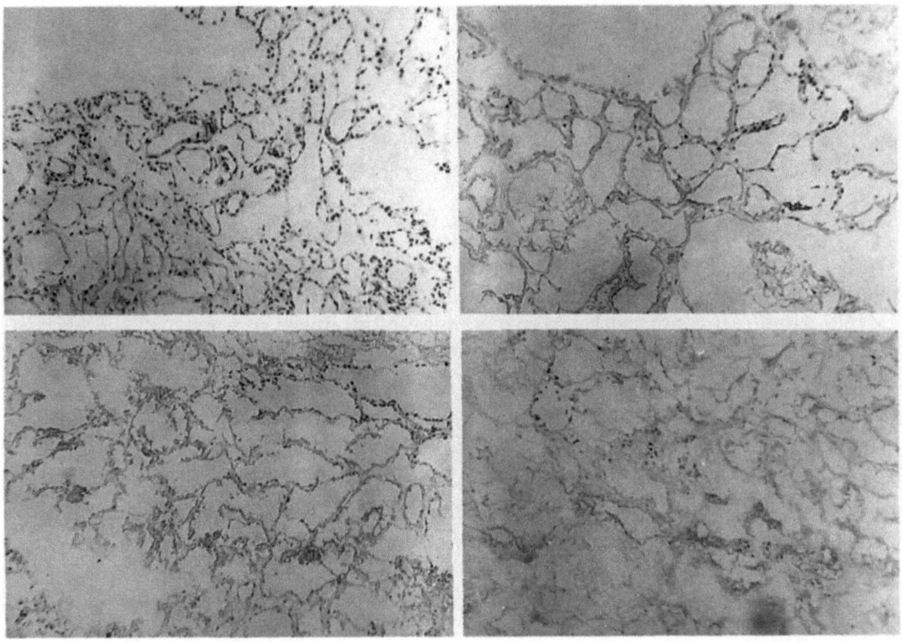

Fig. 2. Immunohistochemical analysis of the expression of c-*fos* (*lower left*), c-*jun* (*lower right*), and *EGR-1* (*upper right*) encoded nuclear proteins in normal renal tissue (×80). Positive staining of nuclei of cells of some proximal tubules. *Upper left*, hematoxylin/eosin staining of a serial section of the same area

tissues were examined. In normal renal tissue a uniform pattern of expression was found; all three gene products were detectable in cells of the proximal tubules only. However, the expression was focal, with not all regions in which proximal tubules were visible expressing the protein. No expression was found in any cells of distal tubules, glomeruli, or collecting ducts. All three genes were expressed coordinately in the described areas (Fig. 2). Consistent with the

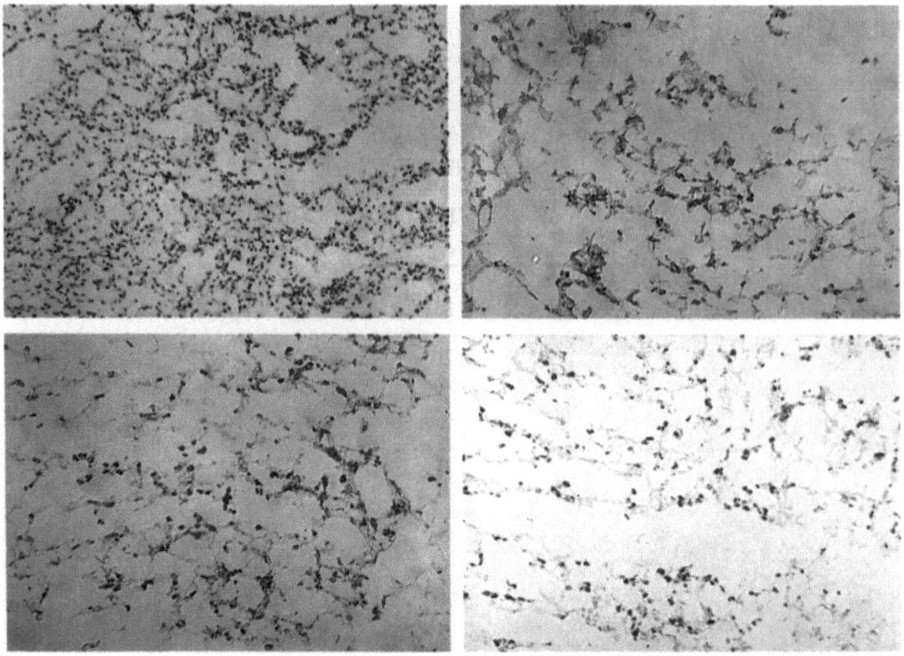

Fig. 3. Immunohistochemical analysis of the expression of the c-*fos* (*lower left*), c-*jun* (*lower right*), and *EGR-1* (*upper right*) encoded nuclear proteins in a renal cell carcinoma (× 160). High expression with positive staining of all nuclei of tumor cells. *Upper left*, hematoxylin/eosin staining of a serial section of the same area (× 80)

transcript data, there was heterogeneous expression of the three early transcription proteins in the eight renal cell carcinomas examined. One tumor did not express any of the three genes; four tumors showed heterogeneous and three homogeneously high expression of c-*fos* and *EGR-1*; three tumors had heterogeneous and two high expression of c-*jun* protein (Figs. 3, 4). Evaluation of the DNA from selected tumor samples showed no amplification or gross rearrangements of any of the three genes as determined by Southern blot analysis (data not shown).

Statistical Analysis. No significant association between gene expression and tumor grade or stage could be demonstrated. After an observation period of 2 years in most of the patients, no significant association with the patient's outcome was found.

Discussion

In this study the role of cellular transcription factors in the development of renal cancer was investigated. The mammalian transcription factor complex AP-1 mediates cellular responses to serum, growth factors, and tumor-promoting

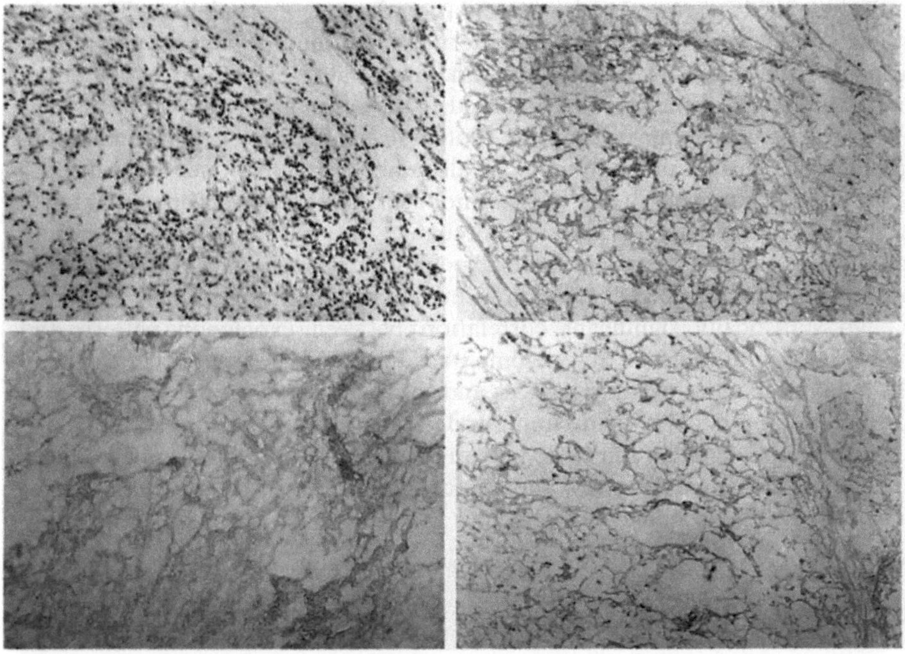

Fig. 4. Immunohistochemical analysis of the expression of the c-*fos* (*lower left*, ×160), c-*jun* (*lower right*, ×80), and *EGR-1* (*upper right*, ×80) encoded nuclear proteins in a renal cell carcinoma. Absent expression with no staining of nuclei of tumor cells. Rarely, single cells appear slightly positive. *Upper left*, hematoxylin/eosin staining of a serial section of the same area (×80)

phorbol esters as well as to the proto-oncogenes c-Ha-*ras*, c-*src*, and c-*mos*. The complex consists of several distinct proteins, including those encoded by the proto-oncogenes c-*jun* and c-*fos* [4]. Disruption of the normal balance between members of the AP-1 complex has been shown to induce malignant cell transformation either through mutations in the coding region or through deregulated expression of normal c-*fos* or c-*jun* proteins [5]. The recently discovered *EGR-1* is highly induced by different mitogenes in a wide array of cell types and belongs into the same class of transcription factors [6, 7].

A heterogeneous expression of all three genes in normal kidney tissue was demonstrated in this investigation. Immunohistochemical analysis revealed that c-*fos*, c-*jun*, and *EGR-1* are expressed only in cells of the proximal tubules. The expression was not uniform, however, in that there were proximal tubules with no expression of these genes. No expression was found in cells of the glomeruli, collecting ducts, or other cells within the normal renal tissue. The detection of transcriptionally highly active cells within normal kidney tissue may be of relevance since it is commonly accepted that renal cell carcinoma arises from cells of the proximal tubules. Another striking phenomenon was the observation that the expression of these genes is coordinate in almost 90% of normal and malignant renal tissues. These results give in vivo support to the theory that immediate early genes may have similar pathways of regulation. The early immediate gene mRNA expression pattern in renal tumors was rather complex. Approximately 20% of the tumors had lower, 40% higher, and 40% equal expression of the genes when compared to its normal corresponding tissues. These results were confirmed on the protein level. The majority of tumors had significant nuclear staining in many or all tumor cells. Only one tumor did not express any of the genes in any of the tumor cells. The absence of any gross DNA alterations in these genes suggests that changes in transcript levels rather than mutation(s) of the genes is responsible for the changes of early immediate transcription factor gene expression in human renal cell carcinomas.

No statistically significant correlation between expression pattern and tumor stage, grade, or patient outcome was found. This however, may be due to the high number of low-stage tumors and the low mortality rate in this cohort. Only 9/47 tumors (21%) had lymph node and/or distant metastases.

The precise contribution of changes in early immediate transcript factor gene expression to the pathogenesis and clinical course of human renal cell tumors remains to be determined.

References

1. Herschman HR (1991) Primary response genes induced by growth factors and tumor promoters. Annu Rev Biochem 60: 281–319
2. Strohmeyer T, Ackermann R (1991) Classic and modern prognostic indicators in renal carcinoma. Urol Int 47: 203–212
3. Sambrook J, Fritsch EF, Maniatis T (1989) Molecular cloning, a laboratory manual, 2nd edn. CSH Laboratory Press, Cold Spring Harbor, chaps 6 and 7
4. Vogt PK, Bos TJ (1990) Oncogenes and transcription factors. Adv Cancer Res 55: 1–35
5. Schütte J, Viallet J, Nau M, Segal S, Fedorko J, Minna J (1989) jun-B inhibits and c-fos stimulates the transforming and trans-activating activities of c-jun. Cell 59: 987–997
6. Sukhatme VP, Kartha S, Toback FG, Taub R, Hoover RG, Tsai-Morris C-H (1987) A novel early growth response gene rapidly induced by fibroblasts, epithelial cell and lymphocye mitogenes. Oncogene Res 1: 343–355
7. Cao X, Koski RA, Gashler A, McKiernan M, Morris CF, Gaffney R, Hay RV, Sukhatme VP (1990) Identification and characterization of the EGR-1 gene product, a DNA-binding zinc finger protein induced by differentiation and growth signals. Mol Cell Biol 10: 1931–1939

Characterization and Functional Significance of the von Hippel-Lindau Gene in Renal Cell Carcinomas

H.-J.H. Decker[1,2], S. Klauck[1], D.I. Smith[3], C. Huber[2], and B. Seizinger[1]

Introduction

The von Hippel-Lindau (VHL) syndrome is an autosomal dominant inherited pleiotropic disorder with virtually complete penetrance and highly variable expressivity. Carriers of the gene have increased susceptibility to a variety of neoplasms of mesodermal and neuroectodermal origin. The most characteristic and frequently observed lesions in VHL are angiomatosis retinae (52%–58%), cerebellar and spinal hemangioblastoma (38%–66%), pheochromocytoma (17%–26%), pancreatic and renal cysts (8%–72% and 25%–60%, respectively; [8] and others). Of those affected by the syndrome, 17%–55% suffer from renal cell carcinoma (RCC), which is one of the most serious and life-threatening complications of the disease. Compared to counterparts with the sporadic form, RCCs in VHL patients occur at an earlier age and are often bilateral or multifocal and are associated with renal cysts. In contrast to simple cysts in the general population, which are usually benign, renal cysts in VHL may contain occult carcinomas. After onset the malignant potential of RCC in VHL is similar to that in the sporadic type, often complicated by metastasis and de novo recurrences. While many VHL patients survive surgery of hemangioblastoma, up to one-third of these patients die of RCC. The incidence of VHL is approximately 1:100000, but it is possible that there are geographic variations, with a regional incidence of 1:40000. There is as yet no sufficient explanation for the primary biochemical defect in VHL or for the variable constellation of tissue type involved in tumor formation. Recent advances in tumor cytogenetics and molecular genetics provide the tools necessary to search for genetic defects in VHL. With the advent of reverse genetics it has become possible to isolate and characterize genes of interest without any hint of their possible functions.

[1] Molecular Neuro-Oncology Laboratory, Massachusetts General Hospital, Harvard Medical School, Boston, MA, USA
[2] Abteilung Hämatologie, III. Medizinische Klinik des Universität, Langenbeckstr. 1 D-55131 Mainz, Germany
[3] Department of Molecular Biology and Genetics, Wayne State University, Detroit, MI, USA

Tumor Studies

Due to improvement in cytogenetic techniques, specific chromosomal aberrations can be described in solid tumors. First clues for the localization of the VHL gene were contributed by cytogenetic studies on RCCs in VHL [2, 8]. Table 1 summarizes the genetic studies in VHL performed so far. Of the RCCs studied 77% have shown involvement of chromosome 3. Loss of a whole chromosome 3, terminal deletions, or unbalanced translocations resulting in partial monosomy of 3p are the most common alterations. The recurrent breakpoints cluster in (3) (p11–p14.2). These findings have been confirmed by molecular studies [3, 10]. Restriction fragment length polymorphism studies have demonstrated loss of heterozygosity in a percentage even higher: 97% of RCCs studied have shown loss of sequences from the chromosome 3p segment.

Applying fluorescence in situ hybridization with single-copy probes from the region of chromosome 3, we have confirmed the loss of DNA sequences from the close vicinity of the VHL locus in RCCs and also in some VHL-associated pheochromocytomas and hemangioblastomas [4]. Torry et al. have determined the parental origin of 3p alleles for six tumors in VHL and found that in all cases deletions of chromosome 3p DNA sequences were from the chromosomes carrying the balancing wild-type allele of the VHL gene [16]. It is very likely that development of tumors in VHL occur through a recessive mechanism analogous to the retinoblastoma model [3].

Linkage, Mapping, and Cloning Studies

Besides somatic changes, RCCs in VHL harbor germline mutations as well. Genetic-linkage analysis with polymorphic DNA markers has been applied as a first step in chromosome-specific cloning techniques for the isolation and

Table 1. Studies of chromosome 3p in von Hippel-Lindau disease

	Involvement	Results	References
Tumor studies			
Cytogenetics	Breakpoints (3) (p11–p14.2)	20/26 RCC 2/10 Pheo 0/8 CH 0/2 AR	2, 4, 8, 10
Molecular genetics	LOH 3p	29/30 RCC 4/6 Pheo 2/4 CH	2–4, 10, 16
Linkage studies	(3) (p25–p26)	55 families	6, 14, 15

RCC, Renal cell carcinoma; Pheo, pheochromocytoma; CH, cerebellar or spinal hemangioblastoma; AR, angiomatosis retinae; LOH, loss of heterozygosity characterization of the VHL gene. We have linked the VHL gene to the locus encoding the RAF1 oncogene [14]. However, the VHL phenotype is not caused by a mutation in the RAF1 gene itself. The localization in 3p25–p26 has been confirmed by other laboratories [6], and others. Despite clinical heterogeneity the VHL locus appears to be unambiguously placed in one chromosomal region by means of linkage analysis. Distinct mutant alleles at the VHL locus may be associated with different tissue specificity. It is also conceivable that the VHL gene locus consists of a complex gene cluster. This question can be addressed once the VHL gene is cloned. We have generated a large number of cosmid probes for chromosome 3. The probes 233E2 (D3S720), 64E2 (D3S719), and 479H4 (D3S719) were characterized and used for linkage analysis. The distance between the flanking markers spans approximately 8 cM. The most likely position of the VHL gene was found to be between RAF1 (centromeric flanking) and 479H4, and 64E2 (telomeric flanking; Fig. 1). 233E2 is the most tightly linked marker for the VHL gene so far identified [15]. It has not yet been

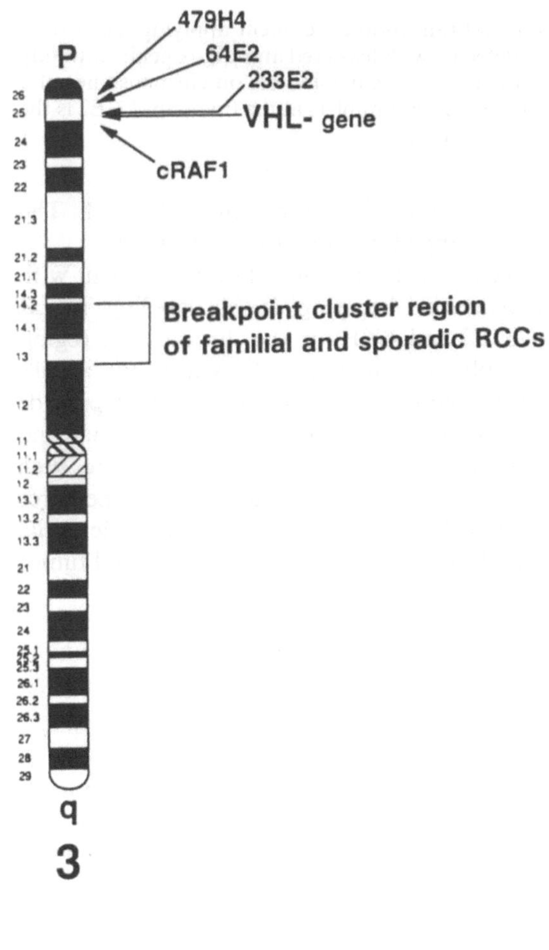

Fig. 1. Chromosome 3 idiogram displaying the localization of our flanking DNA marker, established by genetic linkage, compared to the breakpoint clustering of sporadic and familial RCCs. Note that 233E2 is shown arbitrarily above the VHL locus. It is not possible to establish clearly whether 233E2 maps telomeric or centromeric to the VHL locus

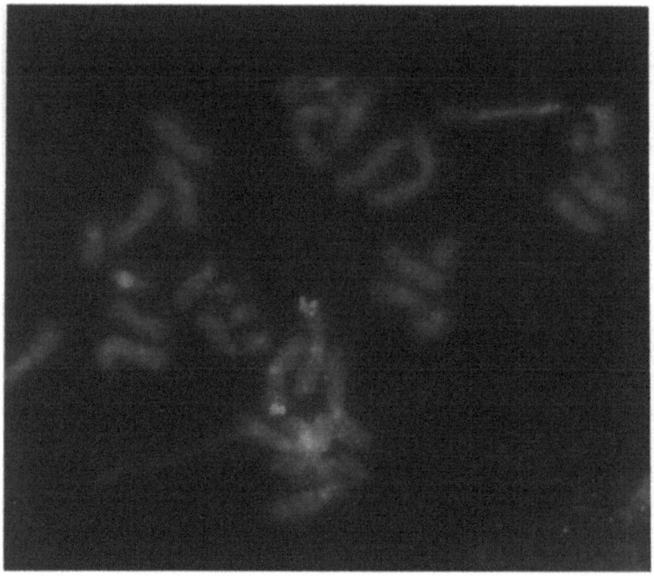

Fig. 2. Fluorescence in situ suppression hybridization experiment applying the cosmid probe 233E2, labeled with digoxigenin, detected with texas red anti-digoxigenin antibody (Boehringer), counterstained with 4′-6-diamino-2-phenylinindiole on chromosomes of a healthy probant. The specific signals are located as doublets at the tip of 3p. 233E2 is the most tightly linked DNA marker for the VHL gene

possible to determine whether 233E2 is telomeric or centromeric to VHL. The probe used for linkage has also been mapped by in situ hybridization.

Figure 2 shows a typical fluorescence in situ hybridization experiment with the probe 233E2 labeled with digoxigenin. Applying double labeling, it was possible to locate the two probes 233E2 and 479H4 in the chromosome region 3p25–p26 [3]. Besides genetic and physical mapping, the search for a submicroscopic deletion in affected family members or in VHL tumors may provide a considerable short-cut for cloning of the gene. Applying conventional and molecular cytogenetics, including fluorescence in situ hybridization, no such deletion has been found yet [4]. Alternative techniques such as VHL pedigree screening for rearrangements by pulsed-field gel electrophoresis or differential hybridization using microdissection libraries and RNA from normal and tumor tissue have also been applied in our effort to clone the VHL gene.[1]

Genetic Testing

Applying the described flanking DNA probes, it became possible to clarify whether individuals at risk are gene carriers or not. Patients with diagnostically ambiguous clinical findings who had a clearly established family history of VHL were identified as not having inherited the defective VHL gene. Depending on the number of probes being informative and the recombination rate of these probes, the error rate of the analysis may be less than 1%. However, a cautious application of this genetic test is recommended until we have gained better insight into the nature of the genetic defect causing VHL [15].

Sporadic Versus Familial RCC

Involvement of the short arm of chromosome 3 in RCC has been described for additional loci proximal to the VHL locus in 3p25–p26: In families with "pure familial RCC" not associated with other VHL symptoms, translocation breakpoints in 3p13–p14.2 have been found. In sporadic RCCs cytogenetic studies have revealed breakpoint clustering in 3p13–p14.2. Restriction fragment length polymorphism analysis has shown loss of heterozygosity in 3p13–p14.2 and in 3p21.3. These findings have lead to the assumption that besides the VHL locus additional loci on 3p may be involved in pathogenesis of familial and/or sporadic RCC. However, this will not be clarified unless the VHL gene (or gene cluster) in 3p25–p26 is isolated and characterized.[1]

Epidemiology

Statistical analysis of age at diagnosis for sporadic and inherited cases of RCC in VHL [12] have provided results similar to those found in retinoblastoma, for example, the age-incidence curves for RCCs in VHL are compatible with a single mutation model, whereas the age-incidence curves for sporadic RCCs suggest a two stage mutation process. These data support the model of the VHL gene functioning as a recessive tumor suppressor gene.

Summary

VHL disease is a hereditary tumor syndrome associated with malignant and benign neoplasias and cysts in multiple organ systems. Of those affected with VHL 17%–55% develop RCC. The expressivity and the age of onset in VHL are highly variable. Despite clinical heterogeneity VHL appears to be linked genetically to a single chromosomal region. We have demonstrated that the VHL gene maps to 3p25–p26. Epidemiologic, genetic, and tumor studies suggest the VHL gene in 3p to function as a recessive tumor suppressor gene. It is feasible that there is more than one gene on 3p centromeric to the VHL locus involved in the carcinogenesis of RCC. Combined genetic approaches are now underway to isolate the VHL gene. The applicability of flanking DNA probes

[1] See also the very recent publication by Latif et al. [11].

for presymptomatic testing in VHL has been demonstrated. The characterization of the VHL gene will be important for understanding of carcinogenesis in RCC in individuals with VHL as well as in the larger number of patients with the sporadic counterparts.

References

1. Bergerheim US, Frisk B, Stellan B, Collins VP, Zech L (1990) del(3p) (p13p21) in renal cell adenoma and del(4p) (p14) in bilateral renal cell carcinoma in two unrelated patients with von Hippel-Lindau disease. Cancer Genet Cytogenet 49: 125–131
2. Decker HJ, Neumann HP, Walter TA, Sandberg AA (1988) 3p involvement in a renal cell carcinoma in von Hippel-Lindau syndrome. Region of tumor breakpoint clustering on 3p. Cancer Genet Cytogenet 33: 59–65
3. Decker HJ, Gemmill RM, Neumann HP, Walter TA, Sandberg AA (1989) Loss of heterozygosity on 3p in a renal cell carcinoma in von Hippel-Lindau syndrome. Cancer Genet Cytogenet 39: 289–293
4. Decker HJ, Klauck SM, Lawrence JB, McNeil J, Smith D, Gemmill RM, Sandberg AA, Neumann HP, Simon B, Green J, Seizinger BR (1993) Cytogenetic and fluorescence in-situ hybridization studies on sporadic and hereditary tumors associated with von Hippel-Lindau syndrome (VHL). Cancer Genet Cytogenet (to be published)
5. Goodman MD, Goodman BK, Lubin MB, Braunstein G, Rotter JL, Schreck RR (1990) Cytogenetic characterization of renal cell carcinoma in von Hippel-Lindau syndrome. Cancer 65: 1150–1154
6. Hosoe S, Brauch H, Latif F, Glenn G, Daniel L, Bale S, Choyke P, Gorin M, Oldfield E, Berman A et al. (1990) Localization of the von Hippel-Lindau disease gene to a small region of chromosome 3. Genomics 8: 634–640
7. Jordan DK, Patil SR, Divelbiss JE, Vemuganti S, Headley C, Waziri MH, Gurll NJ (1990) Cytogenetic abnormalities in tumors of patients with von Hippel-Lindau disease. Cancer Genet Cytogenet 42: 227–241
8. King CR, Schimke RN, Arthur T, Davoren B, Collins D (1987) Proximal 3p deletion in renal cell carcinoma cells from a patient with von Hippel-Lindau disease. Cancer Genet Cytogenet 27: 345–348
9. Kiechle-Schwarz MH, Neumann PH, Decker HJH, Dietrich C, Wullich B, Schempp W (1989) Cytogenetic studies on three pheochromocytomas derived from patients with von Hippel-Lindau syndrome. Hum Genet 82: 127–130
10. Kovacs G, Hsiang-Fu K (1991) Nonhomologous chromatid exchange in hereditary and sporadic renal cell carinomas. Pro Natl Acad Sci USA 88: 194–198
11. Latif F, Tory K, Gnarra J, Masahiro Y, Duh FM, Orcutt ML, Stackhouse T, Kuzmin I, Modi W, Geil L, Schmidt L, Zhou F, Li H, Wei MH, Chen F, Glenn G, Choyke P, Walther MM, Weng Y, Duan DSR, Dean M, Glavac D, Richards FM, Crossey PA, Ferguson-Smith MA, Paslier DL, Chumakov I, Cohen D, Chinault C, Maher E, Linehan WM, Zbar B, Lerman MI (1993) Identification of the von Hippel-Lindau disease tumor suppressor gene. Science 260: 1317–1320
12. Maher ER, Yates JR, Ferguson Smith MA (1990) Statistical analysis of the two stage mutation model in von Hippel-Lindau disease, and in sporadic cerebellar haemangioblastoma and renal cell carcinoma. J Med Genet 27: 311–314
13. Neumann HP (1987) Basic criteria for clinical diagnosis and genetic counselling in von Hippel-Lindau syndrome. Vasa 16: 220–226
14. Seizinger BR, Rouleau GA, Ozelius LJ, Lane AH, Farmer GE, Lamiell JM, Haines JM, Yuen JW, Collins D, Majoor Krakauer D et al. (1988) Von Hippel-Lindau

disease maps to the region of chromosome 3 associated with renal cell carcinoma. Nature 332: 268–269
15. Seizinger BR, Smith DI, Filling-Katz MR, Neumann HP, Green JS, Choyke PL, Anderson KM, Freiman RN, Klauck SM, Whaley JM, Decker HJ et al. (1991) Genetic flanking markers refine diagnostic criteria and provide new insights into the genetics of von Hippel Lindau disease. Proc Natl Acad Sci USA 88: 2864–2868
16. Tory K, Brauch H, Linehan M, Barba D, Oldfield E, Filling Katz M, Seizinger B, Nakamura Y, White R, Marshall FF et al. (1989) Specific genetic change in tumors associated with von Hippel-Lindau disease. J Natl Cancer Inst 81: 1097–1101
17. Vance JM, Small KW, Jones MA, Stajich JM, Yamaoka LH, Roses AD, Hung WY, Pericak Vance MA (1990) Confirmation of linkage in von Hippel-Lindau disease. Genomics 6: 565–567

In Situ Expression of Cytokines in Renal Cell Carcinoma

C. Krüger, I.L. Noronha, H. Stein, and R. Waldherr

Introduction

Cytokines play an important role in the induction and maintenance of specific and nonspecific defense mechanisms by immunocompetent mononuclear cells in malignant tumors, including renal cell carcinoma (RCC) [1, 2]. Cytokines can directly or indirectly influence tumor cell growth and differentiation and are capable of influencing the expression of cell-surface antigens. While examining a series of RCC patients ($n = 20$) by means of immunocytochemistry with a polyclonal antibody to interleukin 6 (IL-6), we constantly observed positive reactions to IL-6 in tumor cells. Similar findings have been reported by other investigators in vitro [5, 8]. It has been suggested that IL-6 functions as an autocrine growth factor in RCC. Furthermore, in vitro experiments have shown that interleukin 4 alone or combined with interferon-γ (INF-γ) or tumor necrosis factor-α (TNF-α) inhibits tumor cell growth and modulates the expression of MHC class I and II antigens in RCC cells [6]. At present, however, only little information is available with respect to the expression of cytokines in RCC in situ. Therefore in a preliminary study we have analyzed the expression of selected cytokines and growth factors in a series of RCC patients by means of immunocytochemistry and molecular biology techniques.

Material and Methods

Material. Tumor tissue from 20 patients (14 men, 6 women; mean age 63 years, range 39–83) with primary RCC was examined. In all patients tumor nephrectomy was performed, and none received any specific treatment prior to nephrectomy. Our series included 17 nonpapillary clear-cell carcinomas and three papillary (chromophilic) carcinomas. Tumor tissue was taken from the periphery of the tumor, avoiding areas of necrosis and degeneration. The tissue was immediately frozen in liquid nitrogen and stored at − 80°C until use.

Pathologisches Institut der Universität, Im Neuenheimer Feld 220/221, D-69120 Heidelberg, Germany

Tumor tissue and normal renal tissue ($n = 5$) were prepared for polymerase chain reaction (PCR), immunocytochemistry, and in situ hybridization.

Polymerase Chain Reaction and Southern Blot Hybridization. Total RNA was isolated using the guanidinium thiocyanate method. One microgram of total RNA was reverse-transcribed into cDNA using either downstream primers or oligo-deoxythymidine. PCR was carried out using specific primers for TNF-α, interleukin-1β (IL-1β), interleukin-2 (IL-2), interleukin-2 receptor (IL-2R), platelet-derived growth factor A (PDGF-A) and B (PDGF-B), platelet-derived growth factor beta receptor (PGDF-βR), and β-actin as control. Each of 40 cycles consisted of a denaturation step of 1 min at 95°C, followed by 1 min annealing at primer-specific temperatures ranging between 52° and 67°C and a primer extension step at 72°C. The PCR products were electrophoresed on a 2% agarose gel in Tris-borate electrophoresis buffer. For further confirmation of PCR product specificity, they were analyzed by Southern blot hybridization. PCR products were blot-transferred onto a nylon-membrane (Schleicher & Schüll/Dassel, Nytran-NY-13N). After transfer the filters were baked at 80°C for 2 h, prehybridized in 10 ml 10 × Denhardt's solution, 6 × SSC, 0.5 mg/ml salmon sperm DNA for 2 h at room temperature, then hybridized overnight in the same buffer containing specific 5'-^{32}P-labeled oligonucleotides. Filters were washed in 6 × SSC, 1% sodium dodecyl sulfate at 60°C and autoradiographed at − 70°C.

Immunocytochemistry. Immunocytochemical reactions were performed with the alkaline phosphatase–anti-alkaline phosphatase (APAAP) method as described elsewhere [9]. The following primary antibodies were used at optimal concentrations: monoclonal antibodies against IL-1β (Genzyme, Cambridge, MA), IL-2 (Oncogene Science, Manhasset, NY, USA), IL-2R (Clonab Tü 69, Biotest Diagnostics, Dreieich, Germany), IFN-γ (Sera-Lab, Crawley Down, UK), TNF-α (CB0006, Celltech, Slough, UK), PDGF-βR (Genzyme), transforming growth factor-β3 (TGF-β3; Oncogene Science), and a polyclonal antibody against PDGF-BB/AB (Genzyme).

In Situ Hybridization. The in situ hybridization procedure was performed as described elsewhere [10] using TNF-α and IL-1β specific antisense riboprobes. The final hybridization mixture contained the ^{35}S-labeled TNF-α and IL-1β riboprobe (2×10^6 cpm/section), 50% formamide, and 1 × Denhardt's solution. Twenty microliters of hybridization mixture was applied to paraformaldehyde fixed cryostat sections and incubated overnight at 55°C in a humid chamber. Following hybridization, the slides were washed in 4 × SSC, 2 × SSC and 1 × SSC at different temperatures. The sections were then dehydrated in graded ethanol and air-dried. Autoradiography was performed by dipping the slides into Kodak-NTB2 nuclear track emulsion at 42°C, under safelight conditions and drying them overnight. The slides were packed in black boxes, stored at + 4°C, and exposed for 5 days. The autoradiograms were developed in Kodak

D19 developer, fixed in Kodak Unifix, and counterstained with hematoxylin-eosin. Negative controls were carried out by hybridizing sections with the corresponding sense probes. In addition, in situ hybridization was performed with sections pretreated with RNase.

Results

Polymerase Chain Reaction. The results obtained by the PCR are summarized in Table 1. PCR analysis demonstrated transcripts of all cytokines, cytokine receptors, and growth factors examined in the majority of tumor specimens (Fig. 1). In particular, we noted transcripts for TNF-α in 90% and for IL-1β in 85% of the tumors examined. This finding was not surprising since we analyzed whole tumor tissue and not isolated tumor cells or short-term tumor cell cultures. These specimens are not only composed of carcinoma cells but also of tumor stroma comprising fibroblasts, mononuclear inflammatory cells, blood vessels, etc. In two cases tumor cell cultures were available from the primary tumors and analyzed by reverse-transcription/PCR. Both cell lines expressed IL-1β and TNF-α.

Immunocytochemistry. The results of the immunocytochemical examinations are summarized in Table 2. Tumor cells and tumor stroma were analyzed separately. IL-1β reactivity (Fig. 2) was observed in 85% of the RCCs, and TNF-α results were positive (Fig. 3) in 70%. Tumor cells exhibited either a diffuse positive reaction within the cytoplasm or a membrane-bound positive reaction. The proportion of positive tumor cells ranged from 5% to 50%. Of note is the fact that only one papillary carcinoma expressed IL-1β (Fig. 2) whereas the other two tumors did not. Similarly, TNF-α was negative in all three papillary tumors. IL-2, IL-2R, and IFN-γ were consistently negative in tumor cells. A few tumor cells expressed PDGF-BB/AB. PDGF-βR, IL-2R, IFN-γ and TNF-α positive mononuclear infiltrating cells were found almost consistently in tumor stroma (Fig. 4) and occasionally interdispersed between tumor cells. PDGF-βR

Table 1. PCR in renal cell carcinomas ($n = 20$)

	n	%
TNF-α	18	90
IL-1β	17	85
IL-2	14	70
IL-2R	15	75
PDGF-A	19	95
PDGF-B	12	60
PDGF-βR	20	100
β-Actin	20	100

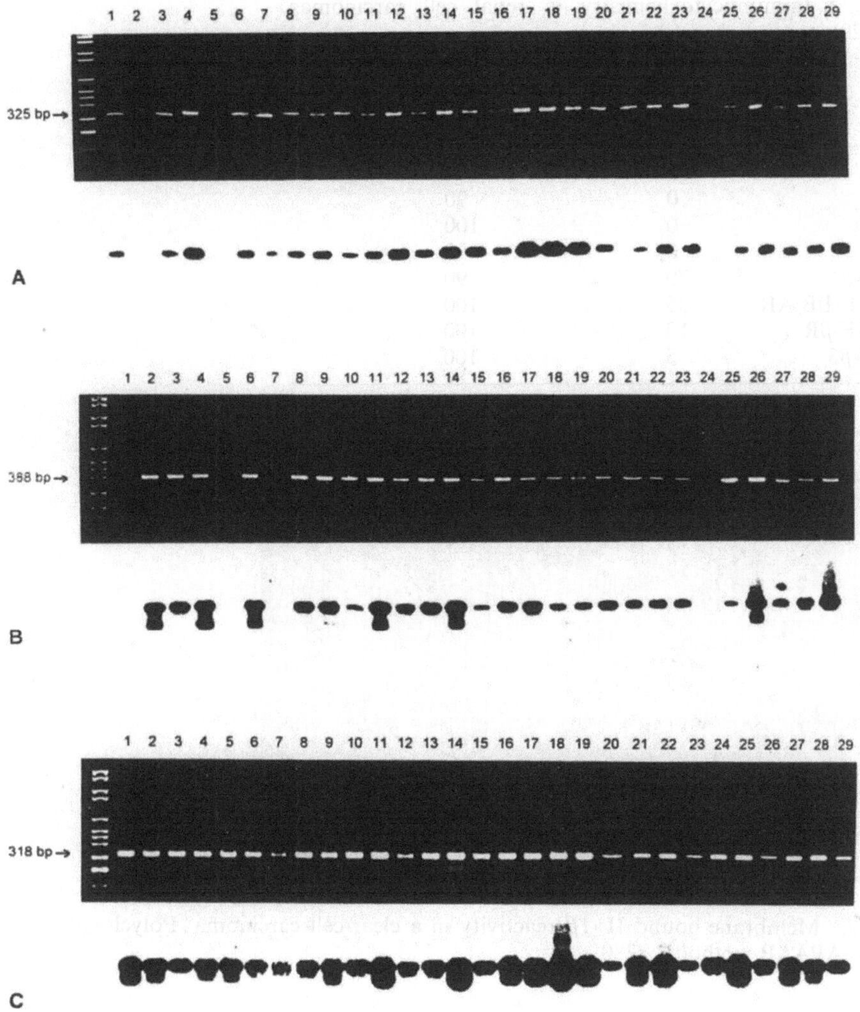

Fig. 1A–C. Agarose gel and Southern blot analysis of PCR products. **A** The TNF-α fragment (325 bp) is expressed in 18/20 tumors (*lanes 1–20*). **B** The IL-1β fragment (388 bp) is expressed in 17/20 tumors (*lanes 1–20*). **C** The β-actin fragment (325 bp) is expressed in all tissues examined. *Lanes 21–27*, positive or negative controls

and TGF-β3 were expressed by stromal fibroblasts and in addition by some mononuclear infiltrating cells.

In Situ Hybridization. To determine whether tumor cells express mRNA for IL-1β and TNF-α in situ hybridization was performed. In 18/20 cases examined a diffuse or focal expression of mRNA for IL-1β and TNF-α (Fig. 5) was observed in tumor cells. In addition, the majority of infiltrating mononuclear cells expressed mRNA for IL-1β and TNF-α.

Table 2. Immunocytochemistry in renal cell carcinomas ($n = 20$)

	Tumor cells %	Tumor stroma %
IL-1β	85	100
IL-2	0	90
IL-2R	0	100
IFN-γ	0	90
TNF-α	70	90
PDGF-BB/AB	35	100
PDGF-βR	10	100
TGF-β3	5	100

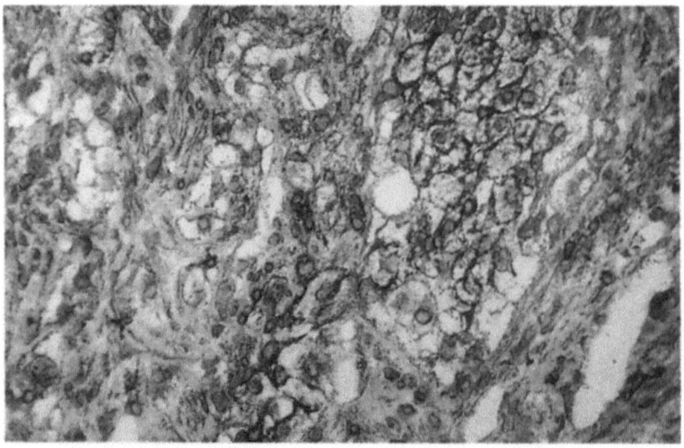

Fig. 2. Membrane-bound IL-1β reactivity in a clear-cell carcinoma. Polyclonal antibody, APAAP method, ×380

Discussion

The results of our preliminary study clearly demonstrate that IL-1β and TNF-α are produced in the majority of nonpapillary RCCs by tumor cells. In situ hybridization confirms the presence of mRNA for IL-1β and TNF-α. The positive reaction at the protein level is documented by immunocytochemistry. The expression of cytokines in cultured carcinoma cells obtained in two of these patients strongly suggests that cytokine expression in carcinoma cells is not an induced but a *constitutive* phenomenon in RCC.

The clinical impact of TNF-α and IL-1β expression in RCCs is unknown. Similar findings have been reported in ovarian cancer [7, 11]. At present we can only speculate on the significance of cytokine production by carcinoma cells.

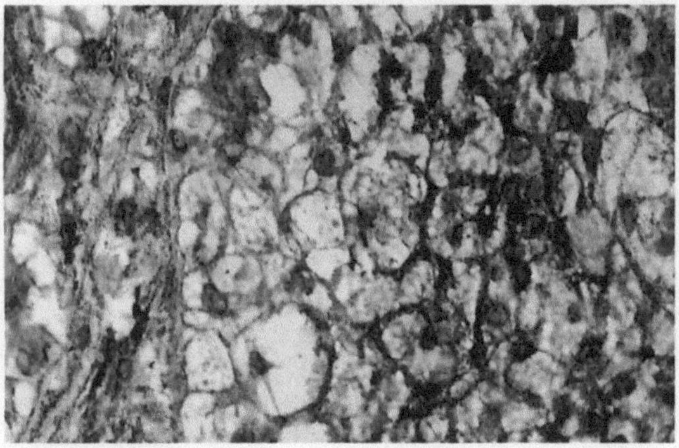

Fig. 3. Expression of TNF-α in a clear-cell carcinoma. Monoclonal antibody, APAAP method, $\times 400$

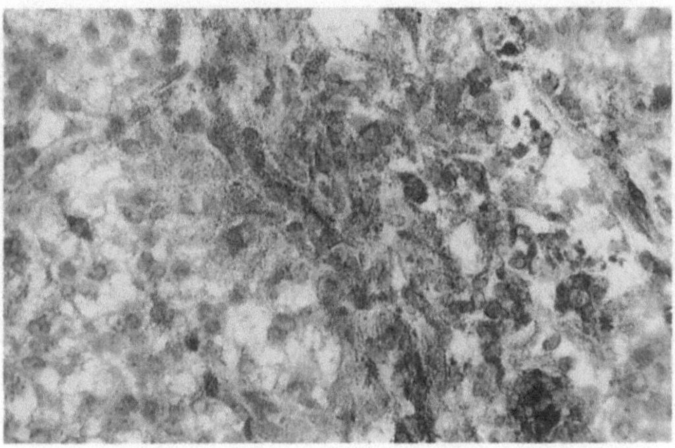

Fig. 4. Mononuclear cells with IL-2 reactivity in the tumor stroma. APAAP method, $\times 380$

Our findings suggest the possibility of a potentially self-perpetuating cytokine induction network in the vicinity of tumor cells. IL-1β and TNF-α production may have either inhibitory or progressing influences on tumor growth [3, 7, 11, 12]. Inhibitory activities could be the result of induction of macrophage-mediated natural killer cell and lymphokine-activated killer cell activity. Furthermore, inhibitory mechanisms could be the result of the production of other cytokines which depress tumor cell growth such as macrophage colony-stimulating factor, IL-6, and monocyte chemotactic protein 1 or a direct cytotoxic effect on tumor cells. On the other hand, TNF-α may enhance the metastatic

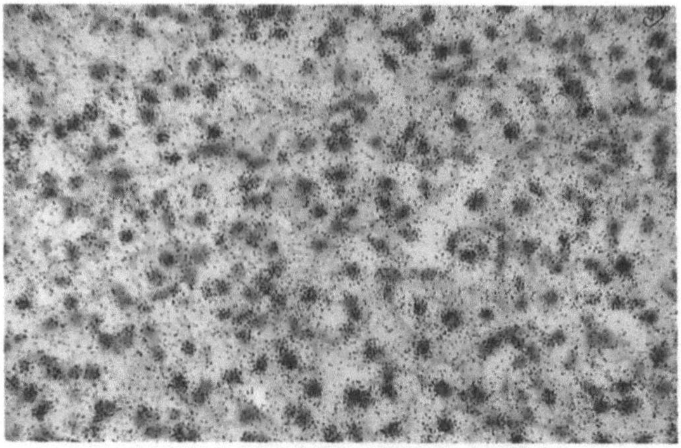

Fig. 5. In situ hybridization (autoradiogram) using a ^{35}S-labeled TNF-α antisense riboprobe. TNF-α mRNA is expressed by tumor cells, $\times 240$

potential of RCCs by an increase in tumor cell adhesion to host cells, the induction of tumor cell metalloproteinases, and stimulation of angiogenesis. It has recently been shown in an in vivo model that low doses of TNF-α induce angiogenesis whereas high doses inhibit the proliferation of microvessels [4]. Thus, local concentrations in neoplastic tissue may be important for angiogenesis. Finally, TNF-α activates several putative oncogenes including c-*jun* [7].

Further studies are necessary to elucidate whether the local production of TNF-α and IL-1β is related to the metastatic capacity and clinical behavior of RCCs.

References

1. Belldegrun A, Kasid A, Uppenkamp M, Topalian SL, Rosenberg SA (1989) Human tumor infiltrating lymphocytes. Analysis of lymphokine mRNA expression and relevance to cancer immunotherapy. J Immunol 142: 4520–4526
2. Belldegrun A, Kasid A, Uppenkamp M, Rosenberg SA (1990) Lymphokine mRNA profile and functional analysis of a human CD4$^+$ clone with unique antitumor specificity isolated from renal cell carcinoma ascitic fluid. Cancer Immunol Immunother 31: 1–10
3. Burrows FJ, Haskard DO, Hart IR, Marshall JF, Selkirk S, Poole S, Thorpe PE (1991) Influence of tumor-derived interleukin 1 on melanoma-endothelial cell interactions in vitro. Cancer Res 51: 4768–4775
4. Fajardo LF, Kwan HH, Kowalski J, Prionas SD, Allison AC (1992) Dual role of tumor necrosis factor-α in angiogenesis. Am J Pathol 140: 539–544
5. Gruss HJ, Brach MA, Mertelsmann, RH, Herrmann F (1991) Interferon-gamma interrupts autocrine growth mediated by endogenous interleukin-6 in renal-cell carcinoma. Int J Cancer 49: 770–773

6. Hoon DSB, Okun E, Banez M, Irie RF, Morton DL (1991) Interleukin 4 alone and with γ-interferon or α-tumor necrosis factor inhibits cell growth and modulates cell surface antigens on human renal cell carcinomas. Cancer Res 51: 5687–5693
7. Malik S, Balkwill F (1991) Epithelial ovarian cancer: a cytokine propelled disease? Br J Cancer 64: 617–620
8. Miki S, Iwano M, Miki Y, Yamamoto M, Tang B, Yokokawa K, Sonoda T, Hirano T, Kishimoto T (1989) Interleukin-6 (IL-6) functions as an in vitro autocrine growth factor in renal cell carcinomas. FEBS Lett 250: 607–6109
9. Noronha IL, Eberlein-Gonska M, Hartley B, Stephens S, Cameron JS, Waldherr R (1992) In situ expression of tumor necrosis factor-alpha, interferon-gamma and interleukin-2 receptors in renal allograft biopsies. Transplantation 54: 1017–1024
10. Noronha IL, Krüger C, Andrassy K, Ritz E, Waldherr R (1993) In situ production of TNF-α, IL-1β and IL-2R in ANCA-positive glomerulonephritis. Kidney Int 43: 682–692
11. Punnonen J, Heinonen P, Kuoppala T, Jansen CT, Punnonen R (1991) Production interleukin-1β and tumor necrosis factor-α in patients with benign or malignant ovarian tumor. J Cancer Res Clin Oncol 117: 587–592
12. Vanhaesebroeck B, Mareel M, van Roy F, Grooten J, Fies W (1991) Expression of the tumor necrosis factor gene in tumor cells correlates with reduced tumorigenicity and reduced invasiveness in vivo. Cancer Res 51: 2229–2238

Tumor-Infiltrating Lymphocytes in Renal Cell Carcinoma: Phenotype, Function, and T-Cell Receptor Usage

O.G. Segurado[1], I. Durinovic-Bello[1], R. Oberneder[2], M. Kriegmair[2], A. Hofstetter[2], G. Riethmüller[1], and D.J. Schendel[1]

Introduction

Several solid tumors, including renal cell carcinoma (RCC), can display pronounced lymphocytic infiltrates which indicate the occurrence of a host antitumor immune response. With the exception of melanoma, the predominant cells that have been cultivated from tumor-infiltrating lymphocytes (TIL) and studied in vitro are nonspecific effector cells [i.e., natural (NK) and lymphokine-activated killers (LAK)] which have been reported to induce a certain degree of tumor regression when adoptively transferred together with high doses of interleukin-2 (IL-2) [4]. In contrast, tumor-infiltrating cytotoxic T-lymphocytes (CTL) displaying specificity for a given tumor have been shown to be 50–100 times more effective [6]. Although immunotherapy with specific CTL might be especially useful in RCC, the in vitro establishment of RCC-specific CTL and definition of the most relevant features allowing them effectively to reduce tumor lesions in vivo are currently not known.

Successful adoptive therapy has been shown to depend on the selection of specific host antitumor T-lymphocytes, on their ability to be recruited in situ, and on the induction of one or several lymphokines in the effector cells [1]. In addition, the cytolytic effect of T lymphocytes on tumor cells seems to be activated mainly through recognition by specific T-cell receptors (TCR) of tumor-associated antigens [5, 14] presented by MHC molecules [2, 6]. Supporting this concept, several studies have shown that MHC polymorphism and bound peptide contribute to the skewness in the TCR gene usage [13], and a similar mechanism has been suggested for RCC-infiltrating T cells [3]. Indeed, recent reports on the TCR gene usage of TIL in melanomas [7] have shown the predominant use of a restricted number of Vα genes. On the other hand, data regarding the phenotypic characterization of TIL and their specificity for MHC-restricted target antigens has not been provided.

In this study we present evidence indicating that TIL bearing characteristic TCR can be isolated from primary tumors of RCC patients. These TIL lyse autologous tumors but do not lyse autologous normal kidney cells and show no

[1] Institut für Immunologie der Universität, Goethestr. 31, D-80336 München, Germany
[2] Urologische Universitätsklinik, Klinikum Großhadern, Marchioninistr. 15, D-81377 München, Germany

or only limited recognition of non-MHC restricted target cells. Furthermore blocking studies with monoclonal antibodies (mAb) reveal an involvement of the MHC and TCR in the TIL-tumor interaction. These results suggest that some RCC display complexes of peptide with MHC which can activate a specific immune response mediated by $CD8^+$CTL.

Materials and Methods

Establishment of TIL Cultures and RCC Cell Lines

Both TIL and RCC lines were established from freshly resected human primary tumors. To establish RCC lines specimens were digested for 4 h at 37°C in RPMI 1640 culture medium containing 0.1% collegenase, 0.002% deoxyribonuclease, and 0.001% hyalurinodase (Sigma, Munich, Germany). Following separation by density gradient centrifugation (Ficoll-Pague, LKB-Pharmacia, Freiburg, Germany) cells from both the interface and the pellet were cultured separately in 75-mm culture flasks in RPMI 1640 medium containing 10% fetal calf serum, 2.5 μg/ml amphoteracin B (Gibco-BRL, Freiburg, Germany) 1% minimal essential medium nonessential amino acids (Gibco), 9 μg/ml insulin (Sigma), 10 μg/ml transferin (Sigma), and 10 ng/ml cholera toxin (Sigma). The same procedure was used to obtain short-term lines of normal renal tissue, obtained at the time of surgery from a site distant from the tumor. For patient 29 an outgrowth of the tumor into the vena cava was also obtained and processed independently. TIL were obtained by cultivating 5-mm pieces of the tumor specimens in 24-well plates in RPMI 1640 medium containing 5% human serum, 10% fetal calf serum, 100 U/ml penicillin, 100 μg/ml streptomycin, 30–50 U/ml recombinant IL-2 (Cetus, Emoryville, CA), and 15% conditioned medium obtained from phytohemagglutinin activated lymphocytes [10]. Peripheral blood lymphocytes (PBL) were used for HLA typing and for TCR repertoire analysis. TIL cultures were fed twice weekly with complete culture medium and split 1:1 as necessary. After approximately 3 weeks adequate numbers of cells were obtained to perform T-cell and NK/LAK phenotyping and TCR analysis. The remaining cells were cryopreserved until the RCC lines were expanded to numbers adequate to allow restimulation of TIL every 10–14 days.

Immunophenotypic Analysis of Effector Cells and RCC Cell Lines

Reactivity to the corresponding surface antigens was analyzed by standard cytofluorometry using single or double staining with murine mAbs specific for CD3, CD4, CD8, CD56, CD57 and HLA class I and II molecules, using local and commercial reagents. For those reagents not directly coupled with fluorescein or phycoerythrin, a fluorescein-conjugated rabbit anti-mouse Ig (Dakopattas, Copenhagen) was used as the second reagent.

Effector Cell Functional Analysis by Cell-Mediated Lysis

Cytotoxicity was measured in a standard 4-h chromium-51 release assay [9] using a panel of target cells which included: autologous normal kidney cells (NKC), autologous RCC lines, and other tumor cell lines, including melanoma (MEL-25), prostate carcinoma (PR-1), the LAK-sensitive cell line Daudi, and the NK sensitive erythroleukemia cell line K562. Inhibition assays were performed by incubating the effector cells with the anti-CD3 antibody (25 μg/ml) or target cells with anti-MHC reagents (ascites diluted at 1:50) for 30 min at room temperature. Subsequently, target or effector cells were added to the wells, and incubation was continued at 37°C for an additional 4-h.

Analysis of the TCR-α and β Repertoire – Molecular Analyses

To analyze the TCR genes utilized by the various effector cells we used a method based on the polymerase chain reaction (PCR) that require minimal quantities of starting material (total RNA) and also allows analysis of in situ TIL. Total RNA was prepared from guanidine isothiocyanate lysates (RNAzol B, Biotecx, USA) of TIL and PBL ($0.5–2 \times 10^6$). The RNA was converted to cDNA using AMV reverse transcriptase (Boehringer Mannheim, Germany) and specific primers for the Cα and Cβ gene segments. This cDNA was then amplified using a battery of oligonucleotides corresponding to 18 previously described TCR Vα and 22 Vβ families, as well as control primers for the constant regions Cα and Cβ. These primers were synthesized, quantitated, and tested for standardization using control PHA phytohemagglutinin-stimulated T cells from healthy donors. As a control of the cDNA synthesis efficiency we determined the amplification level of the V regions as well as from both constant regions of TCR-α and -β using 5′ and 3′ Vα/Vβ consensus primers and Cα/Cβ specific primers, respectively. The specificity of the PCR amplification was assesed by the length of the PCR products and by Southern blotting and hybridization with Cα or Cβ oligonucleotides. Comparative quantitation of each Vα- and Vβ-specific PCR product was achieved using a calibrated quantity of cDNA for each PCR reaction and subsequent computed densitometry of high-resolution gels (Fig. 1). This methodology [11] was used to determine the relative frequency of each TCR gene family.

Cytofluorometric Analyses

The mAbs specific for TCR included reagents detecting Vβ 5.1, 5.2, 5.3, 6.7, 8, and 12 and Vα 2.3 (T Cell Sciences, Boston) and were tested as suggested by the manufacturer.

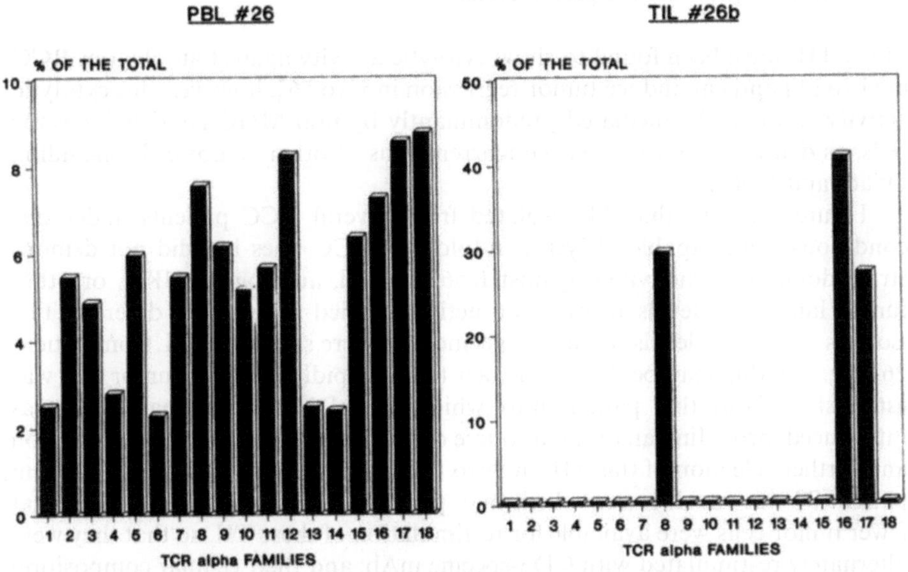

Fig. 1. TCR Vα repertoire analysis: a representative example. Data are presented as the percentage corresponding to each Vα family of the total area, obtained by computer densitometric analysis of the Vα-specific PCR products

Results and Discussion

Cytotoxic T-Cell Lines Can Be Established from In Situ TIL

TIL have been isolated from several patients in numbers adequate for characterization phenotypically, functionally, and for molecular analysis of TCR usage. In two cases reported here autologous tumor lines were available for specificity studies. In vitro outgrowth of in situ TIL was usually obtained within 2–4 weeks. The best conditions for in vitro expansion of TIL were dependent on several factors. Restimulation with autologous tumor cells yielded cultures composed predominantly of T-cells and cultivation in medium with low doses of rIL-2, and conditioned medium enabled isolation of $CD8^+$, CTL. For example, the following phenotypes were found in several TIL populations obtained under these conditions: $CD3^+$ 90.1–99.5%; $CD4^+$ 0.6–11.5%; $CD8^+$ 73–98.7%; $CD56/57^+$ 0.5–3.2%; $TCR\alpha/\beta^+$ 94.2–96.3%. Data are presented as the range of positive cells found in four independently established TIL. These phenotypes contrast with those often reported for TIL isolated from solid tumors following in vitro stimulation with high doses of IL-2 [3] in that they have higher percentages of $CD8^+$ cells and fewer $CD4^+$ cells or cells with markers characteristic of NK and LAK.

Cultured TIL Show RCC-Specific Lysis

Many TIL have been found to show cytolytic activity against autologous RCC in vitro [1] and can induce tumor regression in vivo [6]; however, this cytolytic activity seems to be mediated predominantly by non-MHC restricted effector cells, as demonstrated by their concurrent lysis of other tumor cells, including Daudi and K562.

Figure 2 shows that TIL isolated from several RCC patients under our conditions were capable of lysing autologous RCC lines but did not demonstrate dominant reactivities against K562, Daudi, autologous NKC, or other tumor lines. The levels of cytolytic activity varied among the different TIL isolates. Very high levels of tumor-specific lysis were seen with TIL from patient 26 (Fig. 1a); this may be due to the fact that a rapidly growing tumor line was established from this patient into which the cDNA for human IL-2 was introduced, providing an optimal source of specific antigen for the restimulation and further selection of this TIL in vitro [8]. The cytolytic activity of TIL from patient 29 was much lower, which may partially be explained by the fact that fewer tumor cells were available for restimulation of these TIL so that they were alternately restimulated with CD3-specific mAb, and their cellular composition remained more mixed. TIL 29P (Fig. 1c) was isolated from a miniculture of the primary tumor. Although it showed some lysis of Daudi cells, it did not lyse K562 or autologous NKC; interestingly, the short-term culture of tumor cells from the vena cava outgrowth was poorly recognized. TIL 29C was isolated from a miniculture of the vena cava outgrowth; it too demonstrated a preferential recognition of the primary tumor compared to tumor cells isolated from the outgrowth (Fig. 1d). This difference may indicate that surface changes in the tumor have occurred which alter the interaction with TIL since, as we demonstrate below, the TCR usage is the same in TIL isolates from both regions of the tumor.

The patterns of specificity of these TIL suggested that they contained some effector cells which recognized target antigens on the autologous RCC in an MHC-restricted manner.This could be confirmed for TIL 26 through inhibition experiments using mAbs specific for MHC class I, class II, and CD3 (Fig. 1b). The class I specific reagent W6/32 and a CD3-specific mAb were both able to cause significant levels of inhibition, demonstrating a role for both MHC and the TCR/CD3 complex in the interaction of the TIL with its target. These data suggest that RCC-associated antigens, which most likely represent peptides derived from proteins that are uniquely expressed or overexpressed in RCC compared to NKC, do exist and can induce specific CTL.

TIL Use a Limited TCR Repertoire

If MHC-peptide complexes lead to induction of RCC-specific CTL, it is expected that they would utilize only certain TCR. Thus specific recruitment of

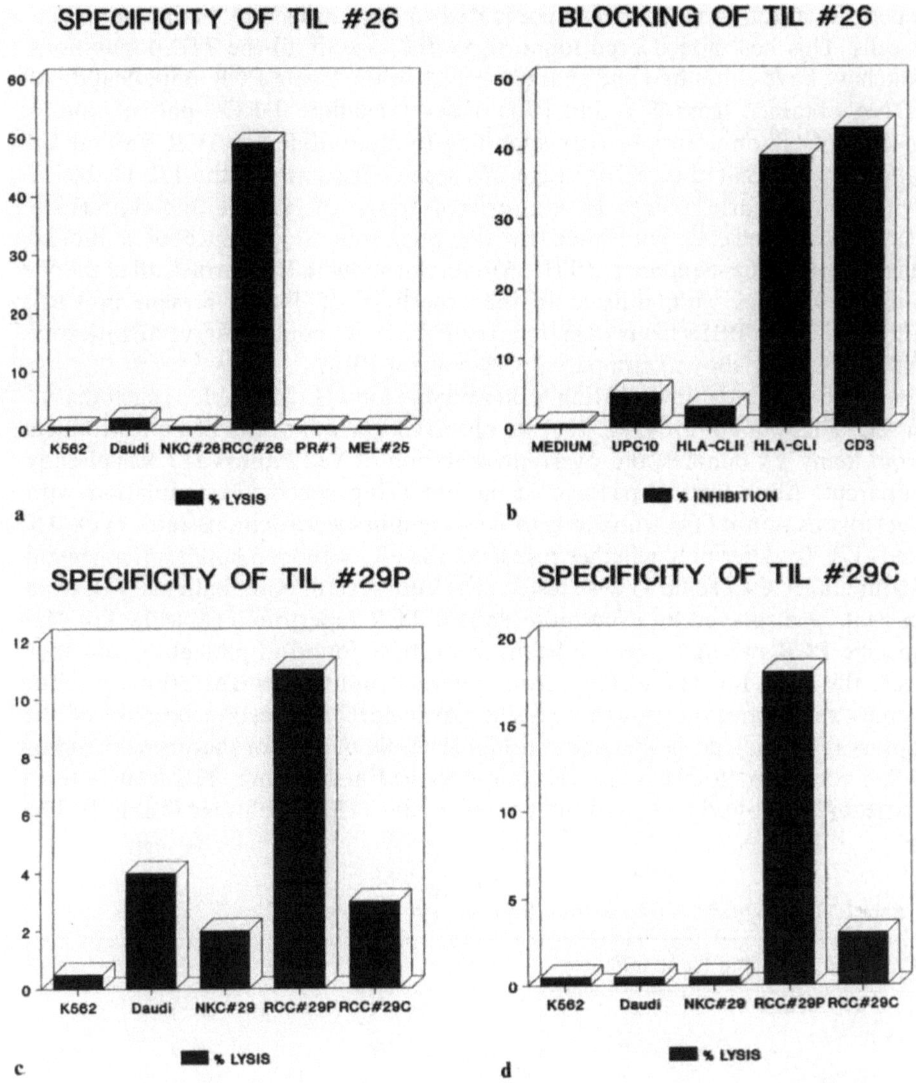

Fig. 2a–d. Analysis of TIL in CML. **a, c, d** The percentage of lysis calculated as follows: (experimental cpm − spontaneous cpm/total cpm − spontaneous cpm) × 100. Spontaneous release was determined by incubating target cells alone in complete medium. Total release was determined by directly counting an aliquot of labeled cells. All percentages were determined using triplicates with single effector to target ratios (E:T) or duplicates with three-step titrations of effector cells. The standard deviations of the replicates were less than 10%. The (E:T) were 4:1 for TIL 26 and 30:1 for TIL 29P and TIL 29C. **b** A percentage of inhibition was calculated as follows: [1 − (% specific lysis with test antibody / % specific lysis with control antibody)] × 100. The percentage of lysis in the absence of any antibody was 33% (E:T = 5:1)

T-cells to the tumor site would be revealed by usage of only a limited TCR repertoire among the TIL when compared to that utilized by peripheral blood T-cells. This has indeed been found to be the case in all the TIL populations which we have cultivated and characterized to date. Using PCR amplification of cDNA obtained from TIL and PBL of several different RCC patients and a battery of oligonucleotides corresponding to many different TCR Vα and Vβ families, very limited receptor usage was seen consistently in the TIL (Table 1). This result clearly points to a restricted usage of VαNJα and VβNDβJβ rearranged genes, as supported by the predominant presence of a limited number of TCRα sequences in TIL 26 (data not shown). In contrast, all of the Vα and Vβ families were utilized in the repertoire of T-cells present in PBL, although in the PBLs from 26 and particularly 29 we could observe quantitative differences (not shown) compared with control PBL.

Some sequential information was available for TIL 26 (Table 1) such that at earlier stages of culture (TIL 26a) we observed low quantities of PCR products from many Vα families, but overrepresentation of Vα12 and Vα17 was already apparent. After further passage in culture using specific restimulation with autologous tumor (TIL 26b), only three Vα families were demonstrated (Vα8,-16, and -17). To determine whether restricted use of Vα and Vβ families is a general feature of RCC-specific TIL we tested cells from several other patients. TIL from patient 29 displayed an even more limited TCR repertoire (Table 1). The Vα-specific PCR products were different from those found in patient 26, but they were the same for TIL isolated from different tumor sites (i.e., primary tumor versus vena cava outgrowth). This is particularly interesting because of the observation that both TIL showed higher levels of lysis of the primary tumor when compared to the vena cava outgrowth. Furthermore, TIL from a third patient (25) showed a skewed but characteristic TCR gene usage (Table 1). The

Table 1. TCR Vα and Vβ repertoire from in vitro cultured TIL

Cell lines	Gene families								
TCR Vα									
TIL 25[a]	1	2	4	8	10				
TIL 26a[b]						12	14		17
TIL 26b				8				16	17
TIL 29P[c]				8					
TIL 29C				8					
TCR Vβ									
TIL 29P	1			8					
TIL 29C				8					

[a] FACS analysis of TIL 25 with a Vα2.3 mAb confirmed the higher frequency of Vα2.
[b] TIL 26a and 26b represent early (< 2 months) and late (> 6 months) stages of the same TIL culture.
[c] TIL 29P were obtained from the primary tumor, whereas TIL 29C were obtained from a tumor outgrowth in the vena cava.

dominant usage of Vα2 in these TIL, as defined by the molecular analysis, was confirmed by cytofluorometric analyses using a mAb specific for Vα2.3. We found increased numbers of cells in three independent TIL isolates obtained from different minicultures which were carried in cultured for 3–4 weeks which stained with this mAb (13%, 11%, and 25%, respectively) whereas positive staining was barely observed in PBL (0.3%).

A recent study has shown that a limited TCR repertoire found in situ corresponds to the predominant TCR sequences from cloned TIL obtained by culturing a virally induced tumor [12]. This also seems to apply to RCC, as demonstrated by the preliminary studies of three patients. In contrast, TCR gene rearrangement studies using restricting fragment polymorphism analysis and hybridization with Cβ probes have shown a limited heterogeneity of Vβ usage in IL-2 stimulated but not freshly isolated TIL [3]. The extent to which MHC-restricted CTL were characterized by such TCR was not determined. In those patients whom we have studied to date the TIL repertoire is different for each patient, although they seem to share some families, such as Vα8. Much more extensive analysis of RCC patients will be required to assess whether characteristic TCR which are specific for given MHC-peptide complexes can be defined, and whether CTL using similar TCR can be identified in patients sharing MHC alleles.

In conclusion, we provide evidence of the existence at the RCC tumor site of highly specific populations of CTL. When autologous tumor is used for restimulation of TIL, $CD8^+$ populations can be obtained which display MHC-restricted specificity in their recognition of autologous tumor. In the TIL that we have examined to date a limited TCR repertoire has been observed that seems to be quite stable and patient specific. This suggests that specific recruitment of T-cells to the tumor site has occurred, and that MHC-restricted immune responses in the host may be directed against RCC-associated tumor antigens. The identification of TIL that mediate cytotoxicity of RCC cells in a MHC-restricted manner opens the possibility to define the tumor-associated peptides that are presented by the MHC molecules. Such antigens have already been defined in mutagenized tumor cell lines and some human melanomas [14]. Knowledge about RCC-associated peptides should be helpful in understanding the mechanism of effective tumor-specific CTL generation and should contribute to improved strategies for immunotherapy.

Acknowledgments. This work was supported by a grant from the German Bundesministerium für Forschung und Technologie (BEO 21, 0319527A) O.G.S. and I.D.-B. were supported by the Alexander von Humboldt-Stiftung, Germany. We thank Ms. B. Maget and K. Seebart for assistance in these experiments.

References

1. Belldegrun A, Kasid A, Uppenkamp M, Topalian SL, Rosenberg SA (1989) Human tumor infiltrating lymphocytes. Analysis of lymphokine mRNA expression and relevance to cancer immunotherapy. J Immunol 42: 4520–4526

2. Borst J, de Vries E, Spits H, de Vries JE, Boylston AW, Mathews EA (1987) Complexity of T cell receptor recognition sites for defined alloantigens. J Immunol 139: 1952–1959
3. Fishleder AJ, Finke JH, Tubbs R, Bukowsky RM (1990) Induction by interleukin-2 of oligoclonal expansion of cultured tumor-infiltrating lymhocytes. J Natl Cancer Inst 82: 124–128
4. Finke JH, Rayman P, Alexander J, Edinger M, Tubbs RR, Connelly R, Pontes E, Bukowski R (1990) Characterization of the cytolytic activity of $CD4^+$ and $CD8^+$ tumor-infiltrating lymphocytes in human renal cell carcinoma. Cancer Res 50: 2363–2370
5. Hom SS, Topalian SL, Simonis T, Mancini M, Rosenberg SA (1991) Common expression of melanoma tumor-associated antigens recognized by human tumor-infiltrating lymphocytes: analysis by human lymphocyte antigen restriction. J Immunother 10: 153–164
6. Kawakami Y, Zakut R, Topalian SL, Stötter H, Rosenberg SA (1992) Shared human melanoma antigens: recognition by tumor-infiltrating lymphocytes in HLA-A2. 1-transfected melanomas. J Immunol 148: 638–643
7. Nitta T, Oksenberg JR, Rao NA, Steinman L (1990) Predominant expression of T cell receptor Va7 in tumor-infiltrating lymphocytes of uveal melanoma. Science 241: 672–674
8. Schendel DJ, Gansbacher B, Oberneder R, Kriegmair M, Hofstetter A, Riethmüller G, Segurado OG (1993) Tumor-specific lysis of human renal cell carcinomas by tumor-infiltrating lymphocytes I. HLA-A2 restricted recognition of autologous and allogeneic tumor lines. J Immunol 151: 4209–4220
9. Schendel DJ, Wank R, Dupont B (1981) Standardization of the human in vitro cell-mediated lympholysis technique. Tissue Antigens 13: 112–120
10. Schendel DJ, Wank R (1981) Production of human T cell growth factor. Hum Immunol 2: 325–332
11. Segurado OG, Schendel DJ (1993) Identification of predominant T-cell receptor rearrangements by temperature-gradient gel electrophoresis and automated DNA sequencing. Electrophoresis 14: 747–752
12. Suzuki M, Koseki H, Mizutani Y, Kuribayashi K, Kanno M, Taniguchi M (1992) Expansion of murine T cells bearing a unique T cell receptor β-chain in friend virus-induced tumor in situ. J Immunol 148: 2968–2973
13. Vachio MS, Hodes RJ (1990) Selective decreases in T cell receptor V beta expression. Decreased expression of specific V beta families is associated with expression of multiple MHC and non-MHC gene products. J Exp Med 170: 1335–1346
14. Van der Bruggen PC, Travrsari C, Chomez P, Lurquin C, DePlaen E, Van den Eynde B, Knuth A, Boon T (1991) A gene encoding an antigen recognized by cytolytic T lymphocytes on a human melanoma. Science 254: 1643–1647

Immunological Approaches to Reverse Multidrug Resistance: The Concept of Molecular Targeting

G.H. Mickisch*

Introduction

Cytotoxic chemotherapy has achieved some cures in primary tumors and even in metastatic disease that are not amenable to effective treatment by surgery or radiation. However, despite initial responses many tumors eventually fail chemotherapy because classical chemotherapy is inadequate to deal with a large tumor burden in many kinds of cancer, and dose intensification which might lead to better results is often hindered by inherent toxic side effects of present chemotherapeutic agents. In particular, both intrinsic and acquired drug resistance remain major impediments to more effective cancer therapies [1].

A common form of multidrug resistance (MDR) in human cancer results from expression of the *MDR*1 gene that encodes a plasma membrane energy-dependent multidrug efflux pump [2–4], termed P-glycoprotein. Pharmacological intervention aimed at inhibiting this multidrug transporter should improve existing chemotherapy of human cancer. Numerous agents which interfere with the activity of P-glycoprotein such as verapamil have been described [5], and the majority of these appear to be substrates for the transporter which compete with anticancer drugs for their transport [6]. However, inherent and potentially toxic side effects of prototype resistance modifiers limit the clinical usefulness of these drugs [7], and the development of new and better agents has been delayed by the difficulty of introducing valid animal models [8]. Using recombinant DNA technology, a transgenic mouse has been engineered whose bone marrow cells express physiological amounts of P-glycoprotein protecting it from the myelosuppressive effect of chemotherapy [9]. Measurements of peripheral white blood cell counts (WBCs) in these transgenic animals provide a rapid and reliable system to assess bioactivity of agents that reverse MDR [10].

Investigations using the monoclonal antibody MRK16 directed against an external epitope of P-glycoprotein [5, 11] have indicated that MRK16 alone

Laboratory of Molecular Biology, DCBDC, National Cancer Institute, National Institutes of Health, Bethesda, MD 20892, USA
* Current address: Erasmus Universiteit, P.O. Box 1738, NL-3000 DR Rotterdam, The Netherlands

may inhibit cell growth of MDR cell lines in vitro [12]. In addition, studies in athymic mice suggest that concomitant administration of MRK16 can prevent development of tumors resulting from subcutaneous inoculation of drug-resistant ovarian cancer cells, and that subsequent injection of MRK16 can slow growth or even sometimes induce regression of established subcutaneous tumors [13]. The present studies determine the efficacy of MRK16 in overcoming MDR in a well-characterized MDR transgenic mouse system and evaluate new options to improve the potency of this immunological approach to reverse MDR in an intact animal.

Materials and Methods

MDR-Transgenic Mice. The development and characterization of transgenic mice expressing the human *MDR*1 gene in their bone marrow have been reported elsewhere [9, 10]. A plasmid carrying the full-length *MDR*1 cDNA under control of a chicken β-actin promoter was injected into fertilized C57BL/6 × SJL F1 mouse embryos, and these transgenic embryos were implanted in foster mice. After establishing a homozygous line (MDR 39), males were backcrossed to MDR-negative C57BL/ × SJL F1 females to generate heterozygous descendants. The amount of *MDR*1 mRNA in bone marrow cells of MDR heterozygous mice is comparable to that detected in the MDR cell line KB-8-5 [9]. This level of MDR expression corresponds to a 3- to 18-fold resistance depending on the drug used [14]. Immunocytochemical analysis has demonstrated that virtually all of these bone marrow cells contain P-glycoprotein at their membrane surface [15]. In these studies, only 6- to 8-week-old sex-matched litter mates were investigated.

Test Conditions. MRK16 (lot nos. 910131C, 910522C) and MRK16F(ab')$_2$ (lot no. 910405C) were provided by courtesy of Hoechst Japan (Kawagoe City, Japan). The manufacturer had purified MRK16 by protein A affinity chromatography and prepared F(ab')$_2$ fragments by pepsin digestion. Cyclosporin A, verapamil, and etoposide were gifts of Sandoz (Basel, Switzerland), BASF Bioresearch (Cambridge, MA), and Bristol-Myers Squibb (Syracuse, NY), respectively. Taxol was from Developmental Therapeutics (NCI). All other drugs were purchased from Sigma Chemical (St. Louis, MO). The drugs were administered by a single intraperitoneal injection into the lower right quadrant of the abdominal cavity. Drug concentrations were adjusted so that a maximum volume of 400 μl was injected per experiment. Each experiment included a minimum of two animals per group and was repeated at least once. In protocols involving MRK16 the monoclonal antibody was dissolved in 0.01 *M* phosphate buffered saline (PBS) containing 2.5% glycine, 3% sucrose, and 0.1% NaN_3 as additives in accordance with manufacturer's instructions and was given 6 h prior to administration of chemotherapeutic agents and/or other chemosensitizers. Peripheral blood was collected by periorbital bleeding with heparinized microhematocrit capillary tubes (Fisher Scientific, Pittsburgh, PA) and diluted 1:20 (vol/vol) in 3% acetic acid solution for erythrocyte lysis. The refractile, viable WBCs were counted on days 0 (before treatment), 3, 5, and 7 in an ultraplane Neubauer's hemocytometer (Hausser Scientific, Pittsburgh, PA). The differential WBC and an estimate of the number of platelets were obtained by using air-dried whole-blood smears which were exposed for 5 min to modified Wright's stain (Accustain, Sigma), neutralized for 5 min in phosphate buffer (pH 7.2) and washed for 10 min in distilled water. Subsequently, the blood film was analyzed under an oil immersion lens.

Construction and Testing of Immunoconjugates. Pseudomonas exotoxin (PE), purified from the culture medium of *Pseudomonal aeruginosa*, was purchased from Swiss Serum (Berne, Switzerland) PE at 5 mg/ml in 0.2 *M* sodium phosphate buffer (pH 7.0) containing 1 m*M* ethylenediaminetetraacetate (EDTA) was mixed with a 20-fold molar excess of succimidyl-4-(*N*-maleimidomethyl)-cyclohexane-1-carboxylate and incubated at room temperature for 30 min. Protein was separated from the unreacted cross-linker on a PD10 column. Monoclonal antibodies MRK16 or MOPC-21 (Sigma), at 5 mg/ml were mixed with a 20-fold molar excess of 2-iminothiolane hydrochloride in 0.2 *M* sodium phosphate buffer (pH 8.0) containing 1 m*M* EDTA and incubated at 37°C for 1 h. The derivatized antibody was separated from the reactants on a PD10 column. Derivatized antibody and PE were then mixed and incubated at room temperature for 20 h [16]. The resulting immunotoxin, coupled by a thioether bond, was then purified by successive chromatography on MonoQ and TSK250 columns [17]. Sodium dodecyl sulfate polyacrylamide get electrophoresis [18] served to assess purity of the eluates. The major immunotoxin peak consisted of a 1:1 conjugate of antibody and PE, and yields were approximately 14% of the starting materials. Inhibition of protein synthesis was used to measure the activity of immunotoxin on cell lines [16, 17]. Cells were seeded at 1×10^5 cells/ml in 96-well flat-bottomed microplates 24 h prior to addition of immunotoxin. Immunotoxins were diluted with 0.2% human serum albumin in phosphate-buffered saline and incubated at 37°C for 24 h. Cells were then assayed for incorporation of [^{3}H]leucine (New England Nuclear; specific activity 1408 Ci/nmol) as described earlier [16, 17]. The mean values of triplicate wells were expressed as percentage of controls that did not receive immunotoxin. For animal studies, immunotoxins were diluted in phosphate-buffered saline containing 0.2% human serum albumin, adjusted to a final volume of 200 μl, and injected intraperitoneally as described above.

Results

There have been reports suggesting a cytotoxic effect of MRK16 alone in MDR cell cultures as well as in athymic mice bearing subcutaneous MDR tumors [12, 13, 21]. We wished to determine its efficacy in an intact animal expressing a level of the human *MDR*1 gene in bone marrow cells which is approximately equal to that found in drug-resistant tumors in people [19]. The resulting resistance is readily assessed by measuring the total WBC of a transgenic mouse prior to and several days after administration of cytotoxic drugs [9, 20]. Figure 1 (upper panel) demonstrates that a dose of MRK16 as high as 2 mg per 20-g animal does not reverse MDR since there was no decrease in WBC of MDR transgenic mice. Next, the potential property of MRK16 as a chemosensitizer in this novel model was evaluated. The data presented in Fig. 1 indicated that the transgenic mice were resistant to the bone marrow suppressive activity of 10 mg/kg daunomycin, whereas the same dose in normal control mice [9, 10, 20] lowered the WBC by approximately 70% of the pretreatment value. However, injection of MRK16 6 h prior to administration of 10 mg/kg daunomycin led to a dose-dependent circumvention of MDR, and a dose of 2 mg MRK16 to enhance daunomycin chemotherapy reduced the WBC by more than 50%. Table 1 summarizes the results with MRK16 plus chemotherapeutic agents from the MDR family of drugs. It is evident that MRK16 reverses resistance against anthracyclines such as daunomycin and doxorubicin, vinca alkaloids such as vincristine and vinblastine, epipodophyllotoxins such as etoposide, and taxol. In addition, MRK16F(ab′)$_2$ fragments displayed a similar ability to overcome MDR in vivo compared to the intact MRK16 antibody (Table 1, right column). This is of potential clinical interest since F(ab′)$_2$ fragments are less immunogenic and may penetrate tumors better than intact antibodies.

However, despite these encouraging results, it was observed that the efficacy of MRK16 as a chemosensitizer is inferior to chemical compounds such as verapamil, cyclosporin A, dihydropyridines, quinine, and quinidine which have previously been investigated in this transgenic bioassay [8, 10, 15, 20]. These drugs induce a fall in the WBC of MDR transgenic mice by chemotherapeutic agents that is equivalent to the drop seen in non-MDR mice given chemotherapy alone. Thus, other options to improve the potency of MRK16-enhanced toxicity to MDR cells were explored.

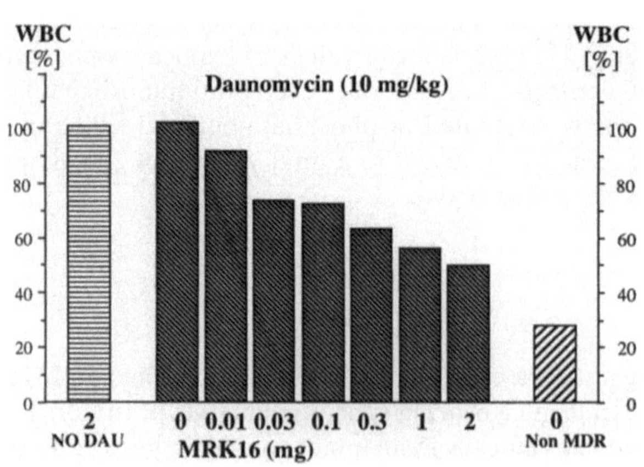

Fig. 1. Efficacy of MRK16 in reversing daunomycin chemoresistance in MDR transgenic mice. Monoclonal antibodies were administered 6 h prior to injection of 10 mg/kg daunomycin, and WBCs were performed on days 0 (before treatment), 3, 5, and 7. Values are expressed as percentage of remaining WBC on day 5 as compared to original value. Non-MDR, normal control mice

Table 1. Reversal of multidrug resistance of MRK16 and MRK16 F(ab')$_2$ in MDR transgenic mice

	MRK16				MRK16 F(ab')$_2$
	0 mg (%)	0.3 mg (%)	1 mg (%)	2 mg (%)	(1 mg)
Daunomycin (10 mg/kg)	100	63	56	48	55%
Doxorubicin (10 mg/kg)	100	60	53	46	49%
Vincristine (5 mg/kg)	100	53	46	43	ND
Vinblastine (10 mg/kg)	100	55	54	49	ND
Etoposide (10 mg/kg)	100	65	56	51	ND
Taxol (10 mg/kg)	100	82	75	74	82%

Monoclonal antibodies were administered 6 h prior to injection of chemotherapeutic agents, and WBCs were performed on days 0 (before treatment), 3, 5, and 7. Values were expressed as percentage of remaining WBC on day 5 as compared to original value. ND, not determined.

First, MRK16 was combined with different prototype chemosensitizers. Previous studies have determined that low doses of drugs such as verapamil and quinine [10] or others (G. Mickisch, M.M. Gottensman, I. Pastan, unpublished results), which produce only partial sensitization of the MDR transgenic mice, were fully sensitizing when used in combination. Figure 2 shows that the combination of verapamil and cyclosporin A in conjunction with daunomycin chemotherapy is highly effective in MDR transgenic mice (Fig. 2A). However, MRK16 combined with neither verapamil (Fig. 2B), cyclosporin A (Fig. 2C), quinine (Fig. 2D), nor quinidine (data not shown) exceeded significantly the sensitization against daunomycin of either drug alone.

Finally, the novel concept of selectively targeting and killing cancer cells with toxins directed via antibodies or receptor-binding proteins [22] was evaluated. MRK16 was therefore conjugated to PE using a conjugation method that produces a very stable thioether bond [17, 22], and its usefulness in MDR-cell lines was tested. Figure 3 demonstrates that MDR-KB-V1 cells are highly sensitive to MRK16 PE (IC_{50} = 0.12 pmol/ml), and that this effect is specific since it was blocked by preincubation with excess MRK16 before adding MRK16 PE. These experiments indicate that in a cytotoxicity assay based on tritiated leucine uptake MRK16 coupled to PE by a thioether bond leads to

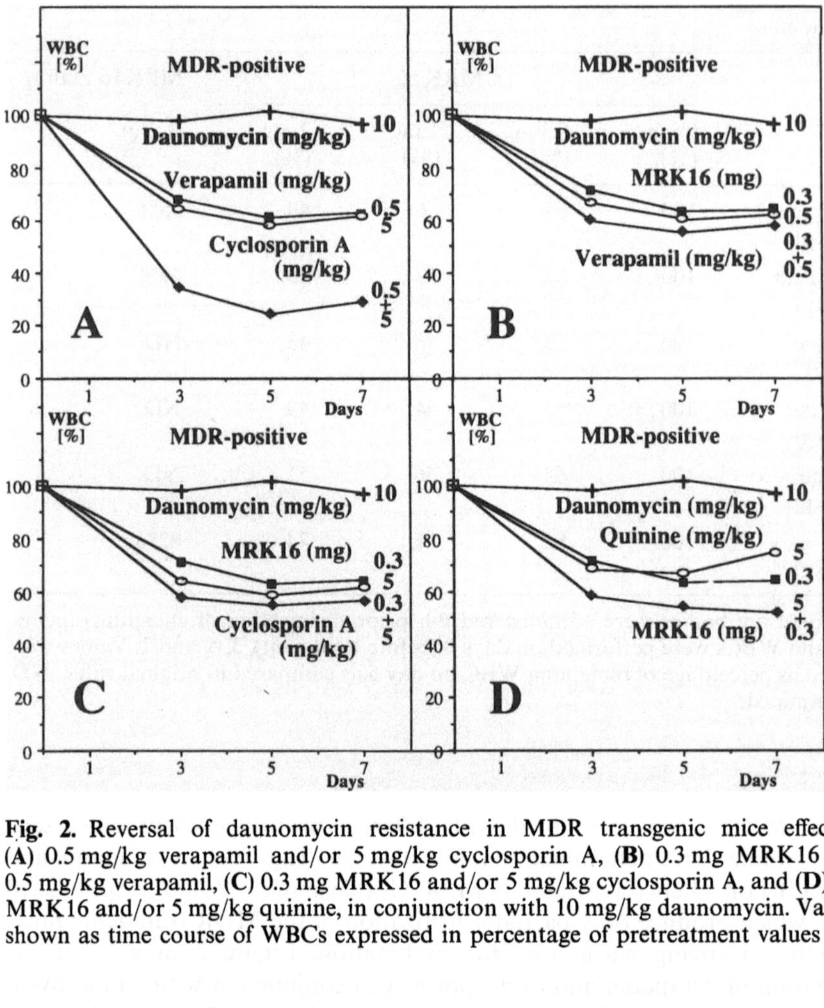

Fig. 2. Reversal of daunomycin resistance in MDR transgenic mice effected by (**A**) 0.5 mg/kg verapamil and/or 5 mg/kg cyclosporin A, (**B**) 0.3 mg MRK16 and/or 0.5 mg/kg verapamil, (**C**) 0.3 mg MRK16 and/or 5 mg/kg cyclosporin A, and (**D**) 0.3 mg MRK16 and/or 5 mg/kg quinine, in conjunction with 10 mg/kg daunomycin. Values are shown as time course of WBCs expressed in percentage of pretreatment values

similar results to those previously reported in which MRK16 was conjugated to PE by disulfide bond and cytotoxicity evaluated by a clonogenic assay [23].

Having established that MRK16 PE is active against cultured cells, we assessed the effect of MRK16 PE in mice. The LD_{50} of MRK16 PE in MDR-negative normal mice was therefore determined; this was 1.5 μg, whereas the LD_{50} in MDR transgenic mice was 4 μg. This appears to indicate that more antigen is available for binding, thus preventing unspecific liver toxicity due to PE [22]. Figure 4 plots the changes in WBC observed after MRK16 PE administration. In normal mice (Fig. 4A) no decrease in WBC was detected. However, in MDR transgenic mice (Fig. 4B) MRK16 PE induced a dose-dependent reduction in WBC by nearly 70%. Figure 4C and D shows control experiments. Injection of excess MRK16 6 h prior to MRK16 PE effectively

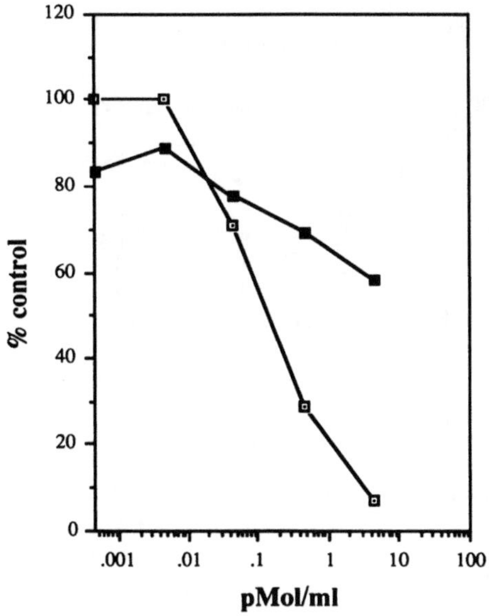

Fig. 3. Effects of MRK16-PE on MDR-cell line KB-V1. Cytotoxicity was measured in a tritiated leucine uptake assay, and values were expressed as percentage of controls that did not receive treatment. —□—, MRK16 PE; —■—, MRK16 (excess) + MRK16 PE

reversed the marrow toxicity (Fig. 4C), MOPC21 is a monoclonal antibody that does not react with human or mouse cells, and MOPC-PE, a non-MDR-related conjugate, did not decrease the WBC of MDR transgenic mice (Fig. 4D). These two results show that MRK16 PE is specifically cytotoxic to P-glycoprotein expressing bone marrow cells in vivo.

Table 2 summarizes the differential WBCs of MDR transgenic mice to reveal cell type specific toxicities of PE conjugates. In addition to the differences in total WBC induced by MOPC PE or MRK16 PE (Fig. 4B, D), the relative distribution of peripheral white blood cells was also affected (Table 2); 0.75 μg MOPC PE did not significantly alter the number or cell type of leukocytes present in blood 5 days after injection of conjugate. Dose escalation to 2 μg led to changes that consisted mainly of an absolute and relative increase in the number of neutrophils, which may be interpreted as signs of unspecific stress reaction. However, MRK16 PE displayed a preferential effect on certain cell types of the differential WBC. At 1 μg, the total WBC was reduced by nearly 50%, but the distribution of cells remained within the range of untreated mice. Higher doses of up to 4 μg further decreased the absolute number of both major types of leukocytes, neutrophils and lymphocytes, but resulted in a relative dominance of lymphocytes. These observations appear to indicate that MRK16 PE acts on MDR bone marrow cells rather than on peripheral leukocytes because specific targeting and killing of precursors of the myeloid lineage in bone marrow would instigate this dramatic and preferential decline of neutrophils after 5 days due to their shorter half-lives compared to cells of the lymphatic lineage.

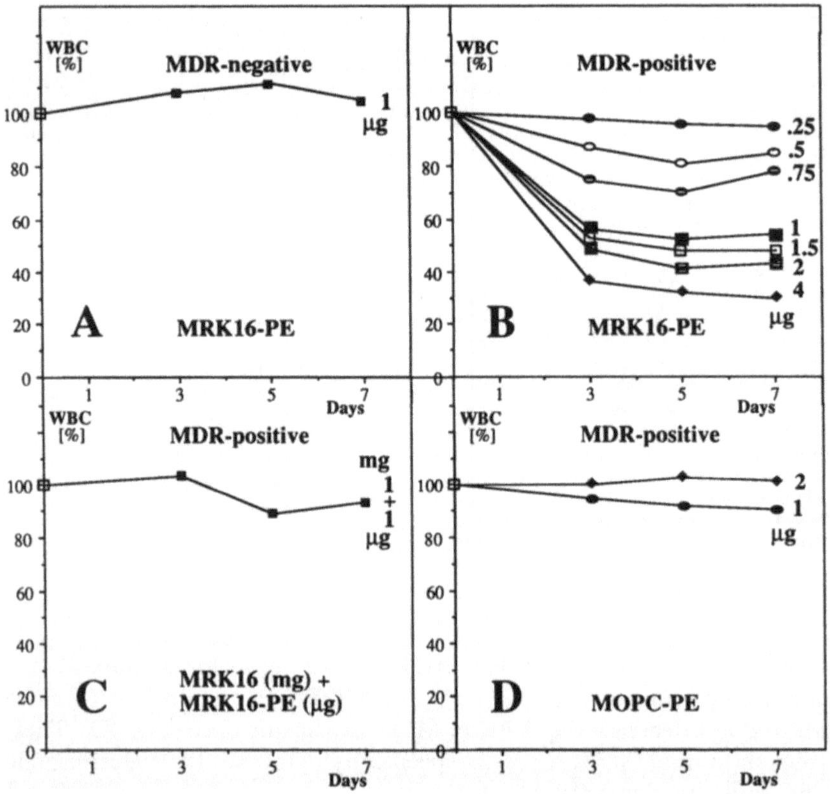

Fig. 4A–D. Effects of *Pseudomonas* exotoxin conjugates on the WBC of mice. **A** MRK16 PE in normal C57BL/6 × SJL mice. **B** MRK16 PE in MDR transgenic C57BL/6 × SJL mice. **C** MRK16 (1 mg) 6 h prior to MRK16 PE (1 µg) in MDR transgenic C57BL/6 × SJL mice. **D** MOPC PE in MDR transgenic C57BL/6 × SJL mice. Values are shown as time course of WBCs expressed as percentage of pretreatment values

Discussion

These studies clearly demonstrate that MRK16 alone does not significantly influence MDR in vivo when bone marrow cells of transgenic mice expressing physiological amounts of the human *MDR*1 gene are used as a parameter (Fig. 1). However, it is obvious that there is a potential for MRK16 and MRK16F(ab')$_2$ fragments as chemosensitizers in conjunction with various chemotherapeutic agents (Table 1). Previous clinical trials have determined that inherent and potentially dangerous side effects of conventional chemosensitizers such as verapamil strictly limit their applicability in humans, and that reduced dosage can achieve only transient tumor responses. Hence, new, better, and less toxic chemosensitizers need to be developed [7, 15]. Given the low toxicity of the immunological approach to reverse MDR described here, these results

Table 2. Differential white blood counts of MDR transgenic mice after injection of *Pseudomonas* exotoxin conjugates

	MRK16 PE				MOPC PE		
	4 μg	2 μg	1.5 μg	1 μg	2 μg	1 μg	0.75 μg
Total WBC ($\times 10^3/mm^3$)	3.3	4.0	4.8	5.3	10.5	9.5	9.3
Neutrophils (%)	0.4 (12)	0.72 (18)	0.48 (10)	1.59 (30)	6.72 (64)	4.5 (47)	3.2 (34)
Lymphocytes (%)	2.8 (86)	3.0 (77)	4.1 (86)	3.7 (69)	3.3 (31)	4.6 (48)	5.3 (57)
Monocytes (%)	0.07 (2)	0.12 (3)	0.19 (4)	0.05 (1)	0.21 (2)	0.2 (2)	0.7 (7)
Eosinophils (%)	–	0.08 (2)	–	–	0.32 (3)	0.29 (3)	0.2 (2)

Differential WBCs were obtained from air-dried whole blood smears 5 days after injection of conjugates. Total WBCs were normalized to $10 \times 10^3/mm^3$, and values are expressed in absolute numbers ($\times 10^3/mm^3$) and as percentage of cells. MRK16 PE, *Pseudomonas* exotoxin coupled to MRK16; MOPC PE, *Pseudomonas* exotoxin coupled to MOPC21.

may lead to come clinical interest, but they also warrant further endeavors to improve the efficacy of MRK16-based chemosensitization (Fig. 1).

Typically, reversal of MDR has been accomplished by exposing drug-resistant cells to alternate substrates for the multidrug transporter which in themselves are not cytotoxic. In tissue culture it has been shown that a wide variety of chemosensitizers circumvent drug resistance by inhibiting the transport of the cytotoxic agent. Thus, elucidation of this mechanism has led to a rational approach for the reversal of drug resistance and the possible treatment of drug resistant cancers [4]. Because chemosensitizers currently in use have specific pharmacological actions of their own as well as a common action on the multidrug transporter, it appears feasible to use them in combination at lower dose levels to overcome drug resistance without producing undesirable side effects. In fact, it has been shown that verapamil and quinine together produce a much greater effect than either drug alone in MDR transgenic mice [10].

The concept is based on the assumption of more than one drug binding site on P-glycoprotein [3, 6] which may lead to differential competition with chemotherapeutic agents when several chemosensitizers are used. MRK16 recognizes external epitopes of P-glycoprotein, and these domains would be implicated in the formation of the putative pore-forming structure of P-glycoprotein [6]. Since drug binding site(s) are believed to be intraplasmatic [3, 5, 6], it appeared worthwhile to address the question of whether combinations of MRK16 with conventional chemosensitizers can act synergistically.

Unfortunately, in an intact animal the combination of MRK16 with various other reversing agents (Fig. 2) did not evoke a more pronounced chemosensitization than either drug alone. Hence, even if a steric hindrance of drug transport is the reason for the chemosensitizing effect of MRK16 (Fig. 1), the allosteric modification of drug binding sites is most likely not responsible for this activity (Fig. 2).

The studies using MRK16 PE proved to be informative (Figs. 3, 4). This anti-P-glycoprotein toxin conjugate specifically and highly efficiently reversed MDR in vitro and in an intact animal. For the time being, several potential uses for MRK16 PE may be anticipated. It may be exploited to purge cell cultures such as bone marrow preparations from MDR cells, and it may serve in an adjuvant setting for the treatment of drug-resistant metastatic disease that remains after surgery or radiation therapy. Thus, this approach of selectively targeting and killing MDR cells appears to merit further attention.

Acknowledgements. This research was supported by the Deutsche Forschungsgemeinschaft (DFG-Mi 334/1-1) and by the Boehringer Mannheim Foundation.

References

1. Pastan I, Gottesman MM (1987) Multiple drug resistance in human cancer. N Engl J Med 316: 1388–1393
2. Kane SE, Pastan I, Gottesman MM (1990) Genetic basis of multidrug resistance of tumor cells. J Bioenerg Biomembr 22: 593–617
3. Endicott JA, Ling V (1989) The biochemistry of P-glycoprotein-mediated multidrug resistance. Annu Rev Biochem 58: 137–171
4. Pastan I, Willingham MC, Gottesman MM (1991) Molecular manipulations of the multidrug transporter: a new role for transgenic mice. FASEB J 5: 2523–2528
5. Tsuruo T (1988) Mechanisms of multidrug resistance and implications for therapy. Jpn J Cancer Res 79: 285–296
6. Gottesman MM, Pastan I (1988) The multidrug transporter, a double-edged sword. J Biol Chem 263: 12163–12166
7. Gottesman MM, Pastan I (1989) Clinical trials of agents that reverse multidrug resistance (editorial). J Clin Oncol 7: 409–411
8. Mickisch GH, Pastan I, Gottesman MM (1991) Multidrug resistant transgenic mice as a novel pharmacologic tool. Bioessays 13: 381–387
9. Galski H, Sullivan M, Willingham MC, Khew-Voon C, Gottesman MM, Pastan I, Merlino GT (1989) Expression of a human multidrug resistance cDNA (MDR-1) in the bone marrow of transgenic mice: resistance to daunomycin induced leukopenia. Mol Cell Biol 9: 4357–4363
10. Mickisch GH, Merlino GT, Galski H, Gottesman MM, Pastan I (1991) Transgenic mice that express the human multidrug resistance gene in bone marrow enable a rapid identification of agents that reverse drug resistance. Proc Natl Acad Sci USA 88: 547–551
11. Sugawara I, Kataoka I, Morishita Y, Hamada H, Tsuruo T, Itoyama S, Mori S (1988) Tissue distribution of P-glycoprotein encoded by a multidrug resistance gene as revealed by a monoclonal antibody, MRK16. Cancer Res 48: 1926–1929
12. Hamada H, Tsuruo T (1986) Functional role for the 170–180 kDa glycoprotein

specific to drug resistant tumor cells revealed by monoclonal antibodies. Proc Natl Acad Sci USA 83: 7785–7789

13. Tsuruo T, Hamada H, Sato S, Heike Y (1989) Inhibition of multidrug-resistant tumor growth in athymic mice by anti-P-glycoprotein monoclonal antibodies. Jpn J Cancer Res 80: 627–631
14. Akiyama S, Cornwell MM, Kuwano M, Pastan I, Gottesman MM (1987) Most drugs that reverse multidrug resistance also inhibit photoaffinity labeling of P-glycoprotein by a vinblastine analog. Mol Pharmacol 33: 144–147
15. Mickisch GH, Licht T, Merlino GT, Gottesman MM, Pastan I (1991) Chemotherapy and chemosensitization of transgenic mice which express the human multidrug resistance gene in bone marrow: efficacy, potency and toxicity. Cancer Res 51: 5417–5424
16. Pai LH, Batra JK, FitzGerald DJ, Willingham MC, Pastan I (1991) Anti-tumor activities of immunotoxins made of monoclonal antibody B3 and various forms of Pseudomonas exotoxin. Proc Natl Acad Sci USA 88: 3358–3362
17. Kondo T, Fitzgerald DJ, Chaudhary VK, Adhya S, Pastan I (1988) J Biol Chem 263: 9470–9475
18. Laemmli UK (1970) Cleavage of structural proteins during the assembly of the head of bacteriophage T4. Nature 227: 680–685
19. Goldstein LJ, Galski H, Fojo A, Willingham MC, Lai S-L, Gazdar A, Pirker R, Green A, Crist W, Brodeur G, Grant C, Lieber M, Cossman J, Gottesman MM, Pastan I (1989) Expression of a multidrug resistance gene in human cancers. J Natl Cancer Inst 81: 116–124
20. Mickisch GH, Merlino GT, Alken PM, Gottesman MM, Pastan I (1991) New potent verapamil derivatives that reverse multidrug resistance in human renal carcinoma cells and in transgenic mice expressing the human *MDR*1 gene. J Urol 146: 447–453
21. Heike Y, Hamada H, Inamura N, Sone S, Ogura T, Tsuruo T (1990) Monoclonal anti-P-glycoprotein antibody-dependent killing of multidrug-resistant tumor cells by human mononuclear cells. Jpn J Cancer Res 81: 1155–1161
22. Pastan I, FitzGerald DJ (1991) Recombinant toxins for cancer treatment. Science 254: 1173–1177
23. FitzGerald DJ, Willingham MC, Cardarelli CO, Hamada H, Tsuruo T, Gottesman MM, Pastan I (1987) A monoclonal antibody-Pseudomonas toxin conjugate that specifically kills multidrug-resistant cells. Proc Natl Acad Sci USA 84: 4288–4292

Therapeutic Applications of Monoclonal Antibodies in Combination with Cytokines in Renal Cell Carcinoma

J. van Dijk, A.J.M.C. Beniers, J.A. Schalken, G.J. Fleuren, and S.O. Warnaar

Immunotherapy with Monoclonal Antibodies

Various murine monoclonal antibodies (mAbs) have been used as "naked" antibodies – not conjugated to radionuclides or toxins – in clinical trials among cancer patients. Although a few complete responses have been observed [1, 2], in general the response rates are low and antitumor effects of short duration. For optimal antitumor activity, mAbs must meet various criteria. First of all, mAbs used for immunotherapy should be specific for antigens present on tumor tissue, preferably with little or no cross-reactivity with normal tissue. For optimal antibody uptake, the tumor must be vascular [3]. The blood supply in large tumors is often deficient, leading to central necrosis and poor uptake of mAb [4]. Apart from these parameters, the size of the mAb-derived immunoreactive component influences the localization pattern in tumor versus normal tissue. Intact IgG has a half-life in patients of approximately 24–72 h, $F(ab')_2$ one of 10–24 h, and Fab′ fragments one of only 1.5–5 h depending on the mAb used [5, 6]. Compared with antibody fragments, intact IgG shows a higher percentage of the injected dose per gram tumor (%ID/g), most probably due to faster clearance from blood of antibody fragments and in the case of Fab′ of reduced affinity [7]. On the other hand, again due to the more rapid clearance from blood, resulting in lower background levels, $F(ab')_2$ and Fab′ fragments have better tumor to blood ratios and therefore show improved tumor imaging [7].

With respect to the antigen recognized, various factors may influence radioimmunoscintigraphy (and therapy). The tumor-associated antigen (TAA) should be present in high density on most tumor cells including the metastases. The mAbs used should have a high affinity for the antigen, as the concentration of mAb near the tumor is low, leading to unfavorable equilibrium binding, especially with low-affinity mAbs [8]. Furthermore, the antigen recognized should be present on the outer membrane of tumor cells. Shedding of antigen into the serum may result in formation of immune complexes, leading to a decrease in injected radiolabeled mAb available for binding to the tumor. Such complexes are known to interfere with localization of the tumor [9]. In contrast

---

Department of Urology, University Hospital Nijmegen, Geert Grooteplain 16, NL-65000 HB Nijmegen, The Netherlands to radioimmunoscintigraphy in which antibody fragments are preferable due to the better penetration into the tumor and because of the more favorable tumor/nontumor ratios, for naked antibody therapy intact IgG is necessary, as the Fc portion is critical for activating the human immune system, for example, in antibody-dependent cellular cytotoxicity mediated by macrophages and/or natural killer cells, or by activation of complement [10–13]. Blocking of the receptors for autocrine growth factors [14] and the induction of host antitumor immune responses, for example, by developing anti-idiotypic antibodies [15], are other mechanisms by which mAbs may elicit anti-antitumor activity. Despite significant numbers of animal studies it is not clear what mechanisms are responsible for the observed regressions of tumors. The somewhat disappointing results of immunotherapy with unlabeled mAbs, mostly of murine origin, may be caused by several factors, such as tumor heterogeneity [16], inadequate delivery of antibody to the tumor [17], or lack of activation of the human immune system. An other major problem associated with the use of murine mAbs is the development of human anti-mouse antibodies (HAMA), which may prevent extended treatment with mAb [18]. The use of human or chimeric mAbs, in which the Fc portion is of human origin and the Fc portion of murine origin, may diminish the antigenicity. However, at present it is not even clear whether the occurrence of HAMA is beneficial or detrimental to the outcome of therapy.

Various experimental studies have shown that mAbs also can be used as a "delivery system" for various toxic agents. Immunoconjugates with toxins derived from plants or bacteria (e.g., ricin, saporin, pokeweed antiviral protein, *Pseudomonas* exotoxin) demonstrate specific antitumor activity in vitro and in vivo against various tumors [19]. Cross-linking of cytotoxic drugs to mAbs also results in potent immunoconjugates and allows targeting of drugs to tumor cells while diminishing toxic drug effects on normal tissue [20]. However, immunoconjugates made with toxin or cytotoxic drugs kill only those tumor cells to which the Mab has bound and subsequently has been internalized. Thus, tumor heterogeneity with respect to antigen expression and internalization rates limits their clinical potential. By using immunoconjugates with radioisotopes, the radiolabel can be localized in relatively high doses to the tumor [21]. A theoretical advantage of radiolabeled as compared to other immunoconjugates is that internalization is not needed, and that radiation damage can be inflicted by "crossfire" to tumor cells not bearing the appropriate antigen. No experimental data exist, however, to demonstrate the effectiveness of crossfire.

Another approach of tumor cell lysis mediated by mAbs can be achieved using bispecific mAbs. Bispecific mAbs combine binding specificities for two different antigens in one molecule. Cytotoxic T lymphocytes normally recognize their target by means of the specificity residing in the T cell receptor. They can, however, be retargeted to recognize other targets with bispecific mAbs. Bispecific mAbs, which bind to tumor cells and to the CD3 antigen which is physically associated with the TCR on T lymphocytes, mediate physical cross-linking between these two cell populations, followed by release of various T cell components, such as pore-forming proteins in close range of the tumor cell which cause tumor cell death [22–27].

Immunotherapy of Renal Cell Carcinoma with Monoclonal Antibodies

Very little data are available on treatment of renal cell carcinoma (RCC) patients with mAbs. In one phase I study 14 patients were treated with escalating doses of up to 25 mg/m^2 with mAb F23 (IgG_{2a}), which is reactive with 90% of RCC. In only one patient, who received 15 mg/m^2 in six does, was a partial response observed in lymph node metastases and lung metastases, with a duration of 17 months. Noteworthy was that all treated patients developed a HAMA response [28].

Several in vitro and in vivo experimental studies indicate that mAbs may have therapeutic potential. By using a mAb, which reacts with a growth-promoting substance, RCC tumor cell outgrowth can be blocked in vitro [29]. Treatment of human RCC, xenografted in nude mice, with anti-RCC mAbs coupled to ^{131}I, resulted in a significant tumor regression or in arrest of tumor growth [30]. Further studies have revealed that small tumors are the most susceptible for antibody-targeted radiotherapy [31]. Furthermore, treatment of tumor-bearing nude mice with anti-RCC mAbs coupled to cytotoxic drug methotrexate results in prolonged survival [32]. The antitumor effect of this immunoconjugate is enhanced by combination with liposome delivery [33].

Biological Response Modifiers

The use of various cytokines in the treatment of RCC seems promising. In RCC patients, interleukin-2 (IL-2), interferons (IFN), and tumor necrosis factor (TNF) have been administered. Clinical trials with IL-2 alone reveal that RCC and melanoma are the most susceptible to treatment, resulting in overall response rates for RCC ranging from 12% to 30% [34–36]. The great variability in response rates observed in various clinical studies may be due to different doses and schedules used. The toxic effects associated with IL-2 limits the use of higher doses of IL-2, known to have better antitumor effect [37].

With IFNs the best responses are observed with certain hematological malignancies, such as hairy cell leukemia [38], but several clinical studies with RCC patients treated with IFNs show a 8%–32% response rate [39, 40]. Complete responses are rare, with relapses occurring after periods of 6 months–2 years. Evaluation of various studies suggests an optimal dosage range for IFN-α, irrespective of treatment schedule [41]. Furthermore, IFN-α seems to give the best results in patients with excellent performance status and pulmonary or nodal involvement only, where tumor burden was minimized by nephrectomy [39].

The mechanisms with which IFNs may exert their antitumor activity are multiple. Experimental data reveal that in addition to direct antiproliferative effects on tumor cells [42], stimulation of the host immune system occurs. This includes stimulation of natural killer cell and monocyte cytotoxicity, for example, by upregulation of Fc receptors, TAA, HLA class I and II antigens, and adhesion molecules [43–45]. Which of these mechanisms actually plays a role is still unclear. It may be relevant that RCC patients with low-stage (stage I or II) disease, treated with IFN-γ show an enhanced infiltrate of $CD3^+CD8^+$ T lymphocytes into the tumors [46].

TNF also has many effects, including direct antiproliferative activity on tumor cells [42]. After binding to TNF-specific receptors on the tumor cell surface, TNF can trigger cell killing due to release of intracellular lysosomal enzymes or production of free radicals [47]. In addition, indirect antitumor effects, related to destruction of the vascular endothelium in the tumor bed have been described [48]. Immunomodulatory functions such as enhancement of macrophage and natural killer cell activity [49, 50], induction of expression of Fc receptors on immune cells [51], and involvement in HLA class I expression have also been ascribed to TNF [52]. However, phase I clinical trials with RCC patients have been disappointing, with only minor responses. The severe toxicity associated with TNF treatment is a major obstacle [53].

Antitumor Effect of mAb G250 in Combination with Interferon and Tumor Necrosis Factor

Earlier in vivo studies have shown that treatment of mice xenografted with human RCC given optimal doses of IFNs in combination with TNF-α results in a complete tumor growth inhibition [54]. However, toxic effect associated with the high doses of IFN and TNF needed for therapeutic effects are a major drawback for human therapy. Some of the immunomodulatory effects induced by IFNs and TNF, as described earlier, such as upregulation of Fc receptors on various immune cells and upregulation of TAA on tumor cells may result in improved antitumor activity over cytokines alone when these cytokines are used in combination with mAbs. In our laboratory a mAb G250 was developed which reacts with 95% of primary RCC and with 86% of metastatic RCC [55]. We tested whether this mAb G250 alone or in combination with IFN and TNF shows antitumor effect on fully established human RCC of significant size in a nude mouse model. We deliberately chose established xenografts and not the so-called Winn-type assay because we felt that the latter is not comparable to the human situation, in which patients often present with fully metastasized disease. Treatment was started 10–14 days after tumor inoculation (tumor size approximately 50 mm^3). The mice were treated subcutaneously peritumoral 3–5 times a week over 6 weeks with various cytokine combinations. Interferons were administered three times a week and rTNF-α five times a week. mAb G250 was given intraperitoneally 3 times a week. The doses used per injection were

150 U/g body weight rIFN-α or rIFN-γ, 30 000 U/g body weight rTNF-α, and 500 μg mAb G250.

Administration of 500 μg mAb G250 per mouse alone resulted in a significant ($p < 0.01$) inhibition of mean tumor growth to 35% of the control group (Fig. 1). Treatment with the doses of rIFN-α/TNF-α or rIFN-γ/TNF-α which have been shown to be optimal for small tumors ($\pm$ 2 mm^3) [54] also resulted in a significant inhibition ($p < 0.001$) of tumor growth to about 35%–45% of the mean size of tumors in the control mice. Treatment with a combination of mAb G250 and rIFN-γ/TNF-α did not result in an enhanced reduction in tumor growth compared to either reagent alone. In contrast, a highly significant further reduction in mean tumor growth was observed for the combination of mAb G250 and rIFN-α/TNF-α compared to either mAb G250 ($p = 0.006$) or rIFN-α/TNF-α ($p < 0.003$ alone; Fig. 1). In this group of ten mice three went into a complete regression. Immunohistochemical analysis clearly showed an enhanced infiltrate of macrophages, which may indicate that apart from the direct antitumor effects of the cytokines also a cellular immune response antibody-dependent cellular cytotoxicity may be important. Striking was the observation that tumors that did not show a complete tumor regression developed progressively growing tumors within 2 weeks after cessation of therapy.

From the preceding it is clear that much remains to be learned about mAb immunotherapy. Whether enhanced stimulation of the immune system as described in tumor models in rodents also occurs in patients with advanced disease, usually selected for phase I/II clinical trials, remaining to be tested.

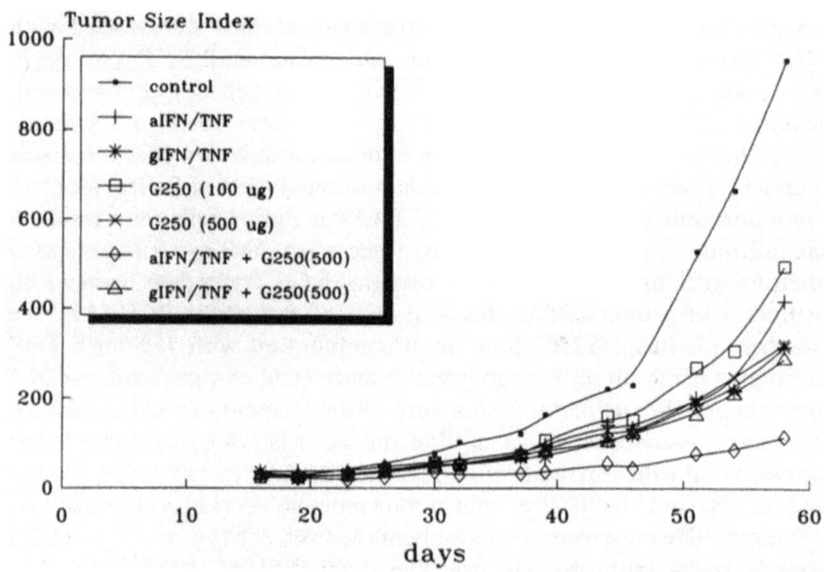

Fig. 1. Effect of mAb G250, rIFN-α/TNF-α, rIFN-γ/TNF-α, and their combination on subcutaneous growth of the NU-12 RCC tumor

However, with respect to RCC the responses obtained even with immunotherapy with cytokines alone are promising. These results, combined with the observation that RCC are often infiltrated with various immune cells such as T lymphocytes and macrophages, suggest that still better responses may be obtained by immunotherapy with combinations of mAbs and cytokines.

References

1. Rosenberg SA, Longo DL, Lotze MT (1987) Principles and applications of biologic therapy. In: DeVita VT Jr, Hellman S. Rosenberg SA (eds) Cancer. Principles and practice of oncology. Lippincott, Philadelphia, pp 301–347
2. Foon KA (1989) Biological response modifiers: the new immunotherapy. Cancer Res 49: 1621–1639
3. Sands H, Jones PL, Shah SA, Palme D, Vessella RL, Gallagher BM (1988) Correlation of vascular permeability and blood flow with monoclonal antibody uptake by human clouser and renal cell xenografts. Cancer Res 48: 188–193
4. Dvorak HF, Nagy JA, Dvorak AM (1991) Structure of solid tumors and their vasculature: implications for therapy with monoclonal antibodies. Cancer Cells 3: 77–85
5. Covell DG, Barbet J, Holton OD, Black CDV, Parker RJ, Weinstein JN (1986) Pharmacokinetics of monoclonal immunoglobulin G_1, $F(ab')_2$ and Fab′ in mice. Cancer Res 46: 3969–3978
6. Fujimori K, Covell DG, Fletcher JE, Weinstein JN (1989) Modeling analysis of the global and microscopic distribution of immunoglobulin G, $F(ab')_2$, and Fab in tumors. Cancer Res 49: 5656–5663
7. Gerretsen M, Quak JJ, Suh JS Van Walsum M, Meijer CJLM, Snow GB, Van Dongen GAM (1991) Superior localisation and imaging of radiolabelled monoclonal antibody E48 $F(ab')_2$ fragment in xenografts of human squamous cell carcinoma of the head and neck and of the vulva as compared to monoclonal antibody E48 IgG. Br J Cancer 63: 37–44
8. Andrew SM, Johnstone RW, Russell SM, McKenzie IFC, Pietersz GA (1990) Comparison of in vitro cell binding characteristics of four monoclonal antibodies and their individual tumor localization properties in mice. Cancer Res 50: 4423–4428
9. Haisma HJ, Goedemans W, Hilgers J (1987) Tumor imaging with monoclonal antibodies. In: Den Otter W, Ruitenberg EJ (eds) Amsterdam, Elsevier, Tumor immunology – mechanisms, diagnosis, therapy pp 23–38
10. Ortaldo JR, Woodhouse CS, Morgan AC, Herberman RB, Cheresh DA, Reisfeld RA (1987) Analysis of effector cells in human antibody-dependent cellular cytotoxicity with murine monoclonal antibodies. J Immunol 138: 3566–3572
11. Lubeck MD. Kimoto Y, Steplewski Z, Koprowski H (1988) Killing of human tumor cell lines by human monocytes and murine monoclonal antibodies. Cell Immunol 111: 107–117
12. Tong AW, Lee JC, Wang R, Ordonez G, Stone MJ (1989) Augmentation of lymphokine-activated killer cell cytotoxicity by monoclonal antibodies against human small cell lung cancer. Cancer Res 49: 4103–4108
13. Pendurthi TK, Parker R, Schlom J, Primus FJ (1990) Lymphokine-activated killer cell cytotoxicity against human colon carcinomas enhanced by monoclonal antibody D612. Int J Cancer 46: 1021–1028
14. Masui H, Moroyama T, Mendelsohn J (1986) Mechanism of antitumor activity for anti-epidermal growth factor receptor monoclonal antibodies with different isotypes. Cancer Res 46: 5592–5598

15. Mittelman A, Kageshita T, Kusama K, Kim JW, Arlin ZA, Ferrone SA (1988) clinical trial of murine antiidiotype monoclonal antibodies to high molecular weig melanoma associated antigens. Proc Am Soc Clin Oncol 7: 248
16. Kerbel RJ (1979) Implications of immunological heterogeneity of tumors. Natu 280: 358–360
17. Jain RK (1987) Transport of molecules in the tumor interstitium: a review. Canc Res 47: 3039–3051
18. Schroff RW, Stevenson HC (1985) Human immune responses to murine monoclo antibodies. In: Foon KA, Morgan AC (eds) Monoclonal antibody therapy of hum cancer. Nijhoff, The Hague, pp 121–138
19. Spitler LE, del Rio M, Khentigan A, Wedel NI, Brophy NA, Miller LL, Harkon WS, Rosendorf LL, Lee HM, Mischak RP, Kawahata RT, Stoudemire JB, Fradk LB, Bautista EE, Scannon PJ (1987) Therapy of patients with malignant melano using a monoclonal antimelanoma antibody-ricin A chain immunotoxin. Cancer F 47: 1717–1723
20. Byers VS, Baldwin RW (1988) Therapeutic strategies with monoclonal antibod and immunoconjugates. Immunology 65: 329–335
21. Order SE, Sleeper AM, Stillwagon GB, Klein JL, Leichner PK (1990) Radiolabel antibodies: results and potential in cancer therapy. Cancer Res 50 [Supp 1011s–1013s
22. Perez P, Titus JA, Lotze MT, Cuttita F, Longo DL, Groves ES, Rabin H, Durda I and Segal DM (1986) Specific lysis of human tumor cells by T cells coated with an T3 crosslinked to anti tumor antibody. J Immunol 137: 2069–2072
23. Lanzavecchia A, Scheidegger D (1987) The use of hybrid hybridomas to tar human cytotoxic T lymphocytes. Eur J Immunol 17: 105–111
24. Titus JA, Garrido MA, Hecht TT, Winkler DF, Wunderlich JR, Segal DM (19 Human T cells targeted with anti-T3 cross-linked to antitumor antibody prev tumor growth in nude mice. J Immunol 138: 4018–4022
25. Van Dijk J, Warnaar SO, van Eendenburg JDH, Thienpont M, Braakman E, Bo JHA, Fleuren GJ, Bolhuis RLH (1989) Induction of tumor-cell lysis by bi-spec monoclonal antibodies recognizing renal-cell carcinoma and CD3 antigen. In Cancer 43: 344–349
26. Van Dijk J, Tsuruo T, Segal DM, Bolhuis RLH, Colognola R, Van de Griend Fleuren GJ, Warnaar SO (1989) Bispecific antibodies reactive with the multidr resistance-related glycoprotein and CD3 induce lysis of multidrug-resistant tun cells. Int J Cancer 44: 738–743
27. Qian J-H, Titus JA, Andrew SM, Mezzanzanica D, Garrido MA, Wunderlich Segal DM (1991) Human peripheral blood lymphocytes targeted with bispec antibodies release cytokines that are essential for inhibiting tumor grow J Immunol 146: 3250–3256
28. Real FX, Bander NH, Cordon-Cardo C, Old LJ, Oettgen HF (1988) Phase I study monoclonal antibody F23 in patients with renal cancer. Proc Am Soc Clin Onco 131
29. Kochevar J (1990) Blockage of autonomous growth of ACHN cells by anti-renal carcinoma monoclonal antibody 5F4. Cancer Res 50: 2968–2972
30. Chiou RK, Vessella RL, Limas A, Shafer RB, Elson MK, Arfman EW, Lange (1988) Monoclonal antibody-targeted radiotherapy of renal cell carcinoma usin nude mouse model. Cancer 61: 1766–1775
31. Chiou RK (1991) The impact of tumor size on the efficacy of monoclonal antibo targeted radiotherapy: studies using a nude mouse model with human renal carcinoma xenografts. J Urol 146: 232–237
32. Sasaki A, Melder RJ, Whiteside TL, Herberman RB, Jain RK (1991) Preferen localization of human adherent lymphokine-activated killer cells in tumor mic circulation. J Natl Cancer Inst 83: 433–437

33. Singh M, Ghose T, Mezei M, Belitsky P (1991) Inhibition of human renal cancer by monoclonal antibody targeted methotrexate-containing liposomes in an ascites tumor model. Cancer Lett 56: 79–102
34. Rosenberg SA (1989) Clinical immunotherapy studies in the Surgery Branch of the U.S. National Cancer Institute: brief review. Cancer Treat Rev 16 [Suppl A]: 115–121
35. West WH (1989) Continuous infusion recombinant interleukin-2 (rIL-2) in adoptive cellular therapy of renal carcinoma and other malignancies. Cancer Treat Rev 16 [Suppl A]: 83–89
36. Bukowski RM, Goodman P, Crawford ED, Sergi JS, Redman BG, Whitehead RP (1990) Phase II trial of high-dose intermittent interleukin-2 in metastatic renal cell carcinoma: a Southwest Oncology Group study. J Natl Cancer Inst 82: 143–146
37. Calabrusi F, Ruggeri EM (1990) Interleukin-2: toxicity and supportive care. Insights Immunother 1: 41–45
38. Quesada JR, Reuben J, Manning JT, Hirsch EM, Gutterman JU (1984) α-Interferon for induction of remission in hairy cell leukemia. N Engl J Med 310: 15–18
39. Muss HB, Costanzi JJ, Leavitt R, Williams RD, Kempf RA, Pollard R, Ozer H, Zkan PJ, Grunberg SM, Mitchel MS, Caponera M, Gavigan M, Ernest ML, Venturi C, Greiner JW, Spiegel RJ (1987) Recombinant alpha interferon: a randomized trial of two routes of administration. J Clin Oncol 5: 286–291
40. Otto U, Schneider AW, Conrad S, Klosterhalfen H (1990) Recombinant alpha-2 or gamma interferon in the treatment of metastatic renal cell carcinoma: results of two phase II/III trails. Prog Clin Biol Res 350: 275–282
41. Krown SE (1987) Interferon treatment of renal cell carcinoma. Cancer 59: 647–651
42. Baisch H, Otto U, Klöppel G (1990) Antiproliferative and cytotoxic effects of single and combined treatment with tumor necrosis factor α and/or α interferon on a human renal cell carcinoma xenotransplanted into nu/nu mice: cell kinetic studies: Cancer Res 50: 3689–3695
43. Lubeck MD, Steplewski Z, Baglia F, Klein MH, Dorrington KJ, Koprowski H (1985) The interaction of murine IgG subclass proteins with human monocyte Fc receptors. J Immunol 135: 1299–1304
44. Weber JS, Rosenberg SA (1988) Modulation of murine tumor major histocompatibility antigens by cytokines in vivo and in vitro. Cancer Res 48: 5818–5824
45. Beniers AJMC, Peelen WP, Debruyne FMJ, Schalken JA (1991) HLA class-I and class-II expression on renal tumor xenografts and the relation to sensitivity for alpha-IFN, gamma-IFN and TNF. Int J Cancer 48: 709–716
46. Onishi T, Machida T, Masuda F, Hatano T, Shirakawa H, Natori T, Hamamoto M, Matsuoka Y (1991) Assessment of tumor-infiltrating lymphocytes, regional lymph node lymphocytes and peripheral blood lymphocytes and their reaction to interferon-gamma in patients with renal carcinoma. Br J Urol 67: 459–466
47. Haranaka K (1988) Tumor necrosis factor. How to improve the antitumor activity and decrease accompanying side effects for therapeutic application. J Biol Response Mod 7: 525–534
48. Palladino MA, Shalaby MR, Kramer SM, Ferraiolo BL, Baughman RA, Deleo AB, Crase D, Marafino B, Aggarwal BB, Figari IS, Liggitt D, Patton JS (1987) Characterization of the antitumor activities of human tumor necrosis factor-α and the comparison with other cytokines: induction of tumor-specific immunity. J Immunol 138: 4023–4032
49. Eisenthal A, Rosenberg SA (1989) The effect of various cytokines on the in vitro induction of antibody-dependent cellular cytotoxicity in murine cells. Enhancement of IL-2-induced ADCC activity by IL-1 and TNF. J Immunol 142: 2307–2313
50. Keller R, Keist R, Wechsler A, Leist TP, Van Der Meide PH (1990) Mechanisms of macrophage-mediated tumor cell killing: a comparative analysis of the role of reactive nitrogen intermediates and tumor necrosis factor. Int J Cancer 46: 682–686

51. Hoffman M, Weinberg JB (1987) Tumor necrosis factor-α induces increased hydrogen peroxide production and Fc receptor expression, but not increased Ia antigen expression by peritoneal macrophages. J Leukoc Biol 42: 704–707
52. Collins T, Lapierre LA, Fiers W, Strominger JL, Polber JS, Recombinant human tumor necrosis factor increases mRNA levels and surface expression on HLA-A,B antigens in vascular endothelial cells and dermal fibroblasts in vitro. Proc Natl Acad Sci USA 83: 446–450
53. Creagan ET, Kovach JS, Moertel CG, Frytak S, Kvols LK (1988) A phase I clinical trial of recombinant human tumor necrosis factor. Cancer 62: 2467–2471
54. Beniers AJMC, Van Moorselaar RJA, Peelen WP, Debruyne FMJ, Schalken JA (1991) Differential sensitivity of renal cell carcinoma xenografts towards therapy with interferon-alpha, interferon-gamma, tumor necrosis factor and their combinations: possible implications for clinical studies. Urol Res
55. Oosterwijk E, Ruiter DJ, Hoedemaeker PhJ, Pauwels EKJ, Jonas U, Zwartendijk J, Warnaar SO (1986) Monoclonal antibody G250 recognizes a determinant present in renal-cell carcinoma and absent from normal kidney. Int J Cancer 38: 489–494

Tools for Vaccination and Immunotherapy: Internal-Image Anti-idiotype Antibodies Resembling the Renal Cell Carcinoma Associated Antigen G250

H. Uemura[1], F.M.J. Debruyne[1], E. Okajima[2], J.A. Schalken[1], and E. Oosterwijk[1]

Introduction

The network concept of the immune system as proposed by Jerne in the early 1970s [1] has gained widespread acceptance. In this concept, the idiotypes of an antibody, defined as the collection of antigenic determinants in the variable region of an antibody molecule, play a major role in the immune response. The antibodies elicited by the variable region (anti-idiotypic antibodies, anti-Id) can be divided into four major types: (a) the anti-Id (Ab2) binds to an epitope remote from the binding site (paratope) of the idiotype antibody (Ab1); (b) Ab2 binds near the paratope of Ab1 and interferes with antigen binding; (c) Ab2 mimics the structure of the antigen recognized by Ab1 (so-called internal-image antibodies); (d) Ab2 recognizes a structure on a constant domain of immunoglobulin (Ig). The potential usefulness of internal-image antibodies to modulate responses to, for example, human tumor-associated antigens (TAA) have stimulated considerable interest in the development and characterization of anti-Id antibodies to these antigenic systems.

However, most human malignancies and spontaneous animal tumors have weak, if any, detectable immunogenic properties, and unequivocal evidence for the existence of unique tumor-specific antigens in human malignancies is still lacking, despite a worldwide extensive search. These observations have led to the conclusion that human cancers are either nonimmunogenic, i.e., do not express tumor-specific antigens, or mediate strong immunoregulatory effects. In this regard renal cell carcinoma (RCC) may be an exception.

The observation of occasional (0.5%–1.0%) spontaneous regression of metastases in RCC patients is suggestive for a host defense mechanism against the tumor [2]. Ritchie et al. have shown that RCC patients have a deficit in T_h cells as well as a decrease in (poorly defined) antibodies against their tumors [3]. T_h cell numbers increase significantly in RCC patients following nephrectomy, whereas with progression of disease the deficit reappears [3]. In addition, Ueda et al. detected a unique RCC antigen in one of 28 RCC examined with autologous typing [4]. These results indicate that RCC patients can raise an

[1] Department of Urology, University Hospital Nijmegen, Geert Grooteplein Zuid 16, NL-6500 HB Nijmegen, The Netherlands
[2] Nara Medical University, 634, Nara, Japan

immune response against as yet unknown target structures present on their tumor.

Since Köhler and Milstein described the production of monoclonal antibodies (mAbs) [5], a number of mAbs recognizing RCC-restricted and RCC-associated antigens have been described [6–11]. Some of the mAbs detect antigens expressed by the tumors only [8, 9], some recognize kidney-differentiation antigens [6–9], and some recognize antigens expressed aberrantly by the tumor cells, i.e., expressed in a restricted number of tissues, but not expressed in normal adult or fetal kidney tissue [10, 11]. The number of unique RCC antigens identified through mAbs is remarkably high in comparison to other tumor types. The fact that RCC is among the most responsive tumors to adoptive cellular therapy may be related to the expression of such unique RCC antigens. Expression of these antigens might be induced by local cytokine production by tumor-infiltrating cells [12]. These unique or aberrantly expressed structures might function as targets in an immune response.

We have raised mAb G250, which reacts specifically with RCC [10]. The G250 antigen is expressed homogeneously in 75% of the RCC examined and is absent from kidney and other normal tissues with the exception of gastric mucosal cells and cells of the larger bile ducts [10]. Animal experiments have shown that mAb G250 can induce complete regression of RCC xenografts [13]. In several mice regression of the RCC xenograft started well after mAb G250 treatment was stopped, suggesting a late antitumor effect. It may be possible that an anti-mAb-G250-Id response was induced in the course of the repeated mAb G250 injections. Based on its restricted expression in normal tissues and the tumor regression observed after mAb G250 treatment in RCC-xenografted mice, we began to isolate and characterize anti-Id mAbs that are true internal-image mAbs, i.e., resemble the RCC antigen recognized by mAb G250 (Fig. 1). Such anti-Id mAbs may be useful in manipulating the immune system of RCC patients.

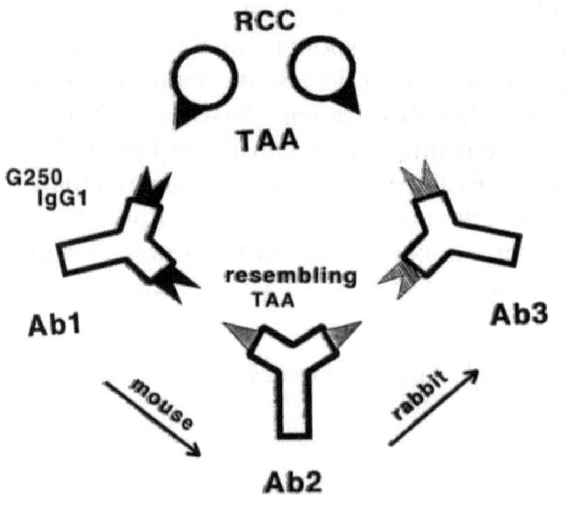

Fig. 1. Production of internal-image antibodies. BALB/c mice were immunized with mAb G250 IgG1(Ab1) cross-linked to Keyhole Limpets hemocyanin. The mice were boosted three times, and splenocytes were fused with Sp2/0 myeloma cells. Hybridomas which produced anti-idiotype antibodies (Ab2) recognizing the combining site of Ab1 (paratope) were isolated. The idiotope of Ab2 resembles RCC TAA, i.e., is the "internal image" of TAA. Rabbits were immunized with Ab2s to investigate whether Ab3 mimicking Ab1 could be induced

Material and Methods

Animals. Eight-week-old Male BALB/c mice were used for immunization and 10-week-old BALB/c nu/nu mice for ascites production. Mice were purchased from the breeding facility of the University of Nijmegen, The Netherlands.

Monoclonal Antibodies. The isolated and characterization of mAb G250 has been described elsewhere [10]. Immunoglobulins were purified by protein A chromatography. $F(ab')_2$ fragments were prepared by pepsin digestion.

Immunization and Fusion. Eight-week-old BALB/c mice were immunized intraperitoneally with mAb G250 IgG1 coupled with Keyhole Limpets Hemocyanin in Freund's complete adjuvant. After three boosters with the same immunogen in Freund's incomplete adjuvant, spleen cells from the mice were fused with mouse Sp2/0 cells.

Screening for Anti-idiotype Antibodies. Hybridoma supernatants were tested by direct enzyme-linked immunosorbent assay for the secretion of Ig (Ab2) reactive with mAb G250 IgG1 $F(ab')_2$ fragments and/or mAb G250 IgG1 $F(ab')_2$ fragments. Cells of positive wells were subcloned on soft agarose and further characterized. Specificity of Ab2s for the combining site (paratope) of mAb G250 was determined by competitive radioimmunoassay and western blotting. In the competitive assay, microtiter wells coated with antigen-positive and antigen-negative cells lysates were incubated with a mixture of serial dilutions of purified Ab2s and a fixed amount of ^{125}I-labeled mAb G250. After washing the binding of the remaining ^{125}I-labeled mAb G250 was measured.

Results

Syngeneic anti-idiotype monoclonal antibodies were generated against mAb G250 (subclass IgG1), a mAb recognizing an RCC-associated antigen. Screening of 4320 wells identified 20 wells that contained hybridomas secreting Ig reacting with mAb G250 $F(ab')_2$ IgG1 fragments. To determine whether these hybridomas recognize the binding site of mAb G250 or the C_H2 region of IgG1, their reactivity against mAb G250 $F(ab')_2$ fragments obtained from mAb G250 IgG1 and IgG2a was investigated. Ten hybridomas showed specific binding to both mAb G250 $F(ab')_2$ fragments. Control experiments with isotype-matched non-relevant IgG1 were negative. Of these hybridomas nine, designated NUH1–9, were subcloned three times on low melting agarose and further investigated. Since idiotypes may be present on the isolated heavy or light chains of Ig, i.e., induce non-internal-image antibodies, western blots of reduced and nonreduced mAb G250 [whole Ig or $F(ab')_2$] and MOPC21 Ig (control) were probed with NUH1–9. Clear staining of nonreduced mAb G250 [IgG as well as

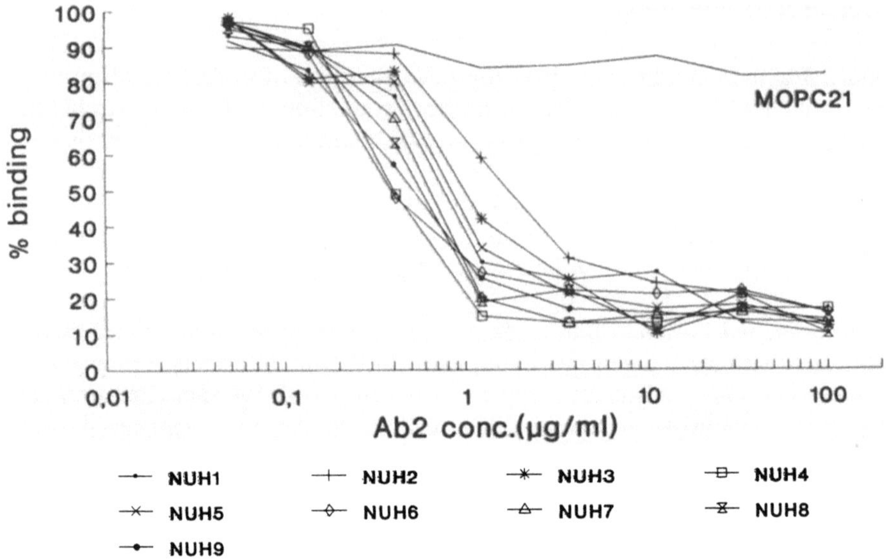

Fig. 2. Competitive radioimmunoassay. mAb G250 was labeled with ^{125}I by the chloramine T method. The immunoreactivity was checked by absorption to G250 antigen^{+} and G250 antigen^{-} cell pellets and ranged between 65% and 85%. Inhibition of mAb G250 binding to G250 antigen was investigated on microtiter plates coated with antigen-positive cell lysates. These were incubated with ^{125}I-labeled mAb G250 at 50% of maximum binding and serial dilutions of Ab2s. After washing binding of ^{125}I-labeled mAb G250 to antigen was measured

F(ab')$_2$] but not of control Ig was observed, whereas no reactivity was seen with the isolated heavy or light chains under reduced conditions (results not shown).

All nine anti-G250-Id mAbs showed a dose-dependent inhibition of ^{125}I-labeled mAb G250 binding to G250 antigen (Fig. 2). NUH4, 6, 8, and 9, required lower concentrations to produce 50% inhibition of ^{125}I-labeled mAb G250 binding to G250 antigen. No inhibition was observed when isotype-matched control Ig was used (Fig. 2). These results strongly suggest that NUH1–9 are internal-image mAbs resembling G250 antigen.

Discussion

Anti-idiotype antibodies (Ab2s) bearing the internal image of a TAA may be used to trigger the host's immune system against tumor cells. Particularly in RCC, anti-idiotype antibodies may be of value because the hosts' immune system seems to play a role in the disease. The first use of passive specific immunomodulation ("vaccination") in cancer patients was immunization with autologous tumor material [14]. Tykka et al. treated stage IV RCC patients with polymerized autologous tumor material and demonstrated a significant improvement in survival [14]. Unfortunately, subsequent studies did not show any benefit for the vaccinated patients [15, 16]. In other tumor types tumor vaccination has been moderately effective.

Recently, several investigators have developed internal-image anti-Id antibodies resembling TAAs [17–23]. Chattopadhyay et al. have investigated an anti-Id mAb mimicking a human high molecular weight melanoma-associated antigen (HMW-MAA) which is expressed by the majority of primary and metastatic melanoma lesions, and by a restricted number of normal tissues [17]. Ab2 administration to rabbits that express HMW-MAA in normal tissues induced anti-anti-idiotype antibodies (Ab3) resembling Ab1, i.e., reacted with HMW-MAA, whereas immunization with HMW-MAA positive melanoma cells did not induce antibodies resembling Ab1. Moreover, some internal-image Ab2 induced Ab3 whereas others did not. These results suggest that subtle differences exist between different internal-image Ab2s, and that expression of a TAA in normal tissues does not suppress induction of Ab3. Subsequent studies have shown that administration of anti-Id resembling HMW-MAA results in a significant longer survival of melanoma patients [24]. The evidence that Ab2s can act as a substitute for a TAA and induce Ab3s functionally resembling Ab1 [17, 21, 24] as well as cellular immune responses [20] shows that anti-Id mAbs may be useful as new therapeutic modality.

The use of anti-Id antibodies as tumor vaccines in clinical trials has been limited. Treatment of melanoma patients with Ab2 mimicking HMW-MAA induced Ab3 resembling Ab1 [23] and prolonged survival [22, 24]. In colorectal cancer humoral as well as cellular responses were observed after the administration of goat or human Ab2 [19–21].

In this communication, we describe the generation and characterization of internal-image anti-Id mAbs resembling a RCC-TAA. We have isolated nine Ab2s (NUH1–9) raised against mAb G250 IgG1 which recognizes an RCC-associated antigen [10]. NUH1–9 all reacted specifically with the variable region of mAb G250 Ab1. In western blots no binding to the separated heavy or light chain of mAb G250 was observed, i.e., the combined heavy and light chains are needed for NUH1–9 binding. These results strongly suggest that all nine Ab2s specifically bind to the combining site of mAb G250 Ab1.

Inhibition experiments show that NUH1–9 all efficiently compete with G250 antigen, indicating that NUH1–9 are internal image anti-Id mAbs, i.e., resemble TAA G250 antigen. All Ab2s show a dose-dependent inhibition of ^{125}I-labeled mAb G250 binding to G250 antigen, but subtle differences were observed. These may reflect different affinities of the Ab2s for mAb G250, resulting in different inhibition curves. Alternatively, they may recognize (partly) overlapping epitopes of the mAb G250 idiotope, i.e., some Ab2s are true internal-image antibodies whereas others recognize a spatially closely located epitope. In the latter case Ab2 binding would result in inhibition of mAb G250 binding by steric hinderance and not because of TAA resemblance. We are performing cross-block experiments as well as binding studies to determine which of these explanations is correct.

We are currently investigating which Ab2s are able to induce Ab3s resembling mAb G250. Preliminary results indicate that some of Ab2s functionally mimic G250 antigen; direct enzyme-linked immunosorbent assays with immune sera from rabbits immunized with NUH1–9 show reactivity with G250 antigen positive cell lysates but not with G250 antigen negative cell lysates (data not shown). We hope that these anti-idiotype mAbs can be used for immunotherapy in RCC patients.

References

1. Jerne NK (1974) Towards a network theory of the immune system. Ann Immunol 125 C: 373–389
2. De Riese W, Allhoff E, Kirchner H et al. (1991) Complete spontaneous regression in metastatic renal cell carcinoma – an update and review. World J Urol 9: 184–191
3. Ritchie AWS, James K, Micklem HS, Chisholm GD (1984) Lymphocyte subsets in renal cell carcinoma – a sequential study using monoclonal antibodies. Br J Urol 56: 140–148
4. Ueda R, Shiku H, Pfeundschuh et al. (1979) Cell surface antigens of human renal cancer defined by autologous typing. J Exp Med 150: 564–579
5. Köhler G, Milstein C (1975) Continuous culture of fused cells secreting antibody of predefined specificity. Nature 265: 495–497
6. Oosterwijk E, Ruiter DJ, Wakka JC et al. (1986) Immunohistochemical analysis of monoclonal antibodies to renal antigens. Am J Pathol 123: 301–309
7. Luner SJ, Ghose T, Chatterjee S et al. (1986) Monoclonal antibodies to kidney and tumor-associated surface antigens of human renal cell carcinoma. Cancer Res 46: 5816–5820
8. Vessella RL, Moon TD, Chiou RK et al. (1985) Monoclonal antibodies to renal cell carcinoma: recognition of shared and restricted tissue antigens. Cancer Res 45: 6131–6139
9. Finstad CL, Cordon-Cardo C, Bander NH et al. (1985) Specificity analysis of mouse monoclonal antibodies defining cell surface antigens of human renal cancer. Proc Natl Acad Sci USA 82: 2955–2959
10. Oosterwijk E, Ruiter DJ, Hoedemaeker PJ et al. (1986) Monoclonal antibody G250 recognizes a determinant present in renal-cell carcinoma and absent from normal kidney. Int J Cancer 38: 489–494
11. Wahlström Y, Närvänen A, Suni J et al. (1985) Mr 75,000 protein, a tumor marker in renal cell adenocarcinoma, reacting with antibodies to a synthetic peptide based on a cloned human endogeneous retroviral nucleotide sequence. Int J Cancer 36: 379–382
12. Haas GP, Pontes JE, Belldegrun A (1992) Tumor infiltrating lymphocytes in renal cell carcinoma. In: Staehler G, Pomer S (eds) Basic and clinical research on renal cell carcinoma. Springer, Berlin Heidelberg New York, pp 200–211
13. Van Dijk J (1991) Renal cell carcinoma: diagnostic and therapeutic applications of monoclonal antibodies. Thesis, University of Leiden, pp 97–113
14. Tykka H, Oravisto KJ, Lehtonen T et al. (1978) Active specific immunotherapy of advanced renal-cell carcinoma. Eur Urol 4: 250–258
15. Fowler JE Jr (1986) Failure of immunotherapy for metastatic renal cell carcinoma. J Urol 135: 22–25
16. Schaerfe T, Mueller S, Riedmiller H et al. (1989) Immunotherapy of metastasizing renal cell carcinoma. Results of multicentered trial. Urol Int 44: 1–4
17. Chattopadhyay P, Kaveri SV, Byars N et al. (1991) Human high molecular weight-

melanoma associated antigen mimicry by an anti-idiotypic antibody: characterization of the immunogenicity and the immune response to the mouse monoclonal antibody IMel-1. Cancer Res 51: 6045–6051
18. Kahn M, Hellström I, Estin CD, Hellström KE (1989) Monoclonal antiidiotypic antibodies related to p97 human melanoma antigen. Cancer Res 49: 3157–3162
19. Robins RA, Denton GWL, Hardcastle JD et al. (1991) Anti-tumor immune response and interleukin-2 production induced in colorectal cancer patients by immunization of human monoclonal anti-idiotype antibody. Cancer Res 51: 5425–5429
20. Mellstedt H, Frödin J-E, Birberfeld P et al. (1991) Patients treated with monoclonal antibody (ab1) to the colorectal carcinoma antigen 17-1A develop a cellular response (DTH) to the "internal image of antigen" (ab2). Int J Cancer 48: 344–349
21. Herlyn D, Wettendorf M, Schmoll E et al. (1987) Anti-idiotype immunization of cancer patients: modulation of the immune response. Proc Natl Acad Sci USA 84: 8055–8059
22. Ferrone S (1990) Monoclonal antibodies and tumor vaccines. Curr Opin Oncol 2: 1146–1151
23. Mittelman A, Chen ZJ, Kageshita T et al. (1990) Active specific immunotherapy in patients with melanoma. J Clin Invest 86: 2136–2144
24. Chen ZJ, Mittelman A, Tang H et al. (1992) Immunotherapy with mouse antiidiotypic mAb in melanoma. Proc AACR 83: 333

Laser Photodynamic Therapy of Xenotransplanted Human Renal Cell Carcinoma

S. Pomer[1], G. Graschew[2], H. Sinn[2], T. Kälble[1], and G. Staehler[1]

Introduction

Photodynamic therapy (PDT) has recently attracted much attention, especially among urologists, because it appears to be a selective form of cancer treatment which causes minimal damage to surrounding normal tissues. In particular, the multifocal bladder carcinoma in situ, up to now difficult to detect endoscopically, has become a new domain for the integral laser photodynamic therapy [1–3].

The purpose of this study was to evaluate laser PDT for its efficacy in destroying renal cell carcinoma. Currently, renal cell carcinoma is usually treated by nephrectomy. Radical nephrectomy with primary control of the renal vessels and regional lymphadenectomy is still considered the standard treatment of renal cell carcinoma. However, the need for excisional parenchyma-sparing surgical procedures is well justified. The nephron-sparing surgery of small peripheral lesions yields excellent results [4, 5] even in the presence of a normal contralateral kidney. The need for nephron-sparing renal surgery has been demonstrated, and it seems that in many cases the complete organ loss with its unfortunate consequence for the patient can be obviated [5, 6]. The widening of the concept of cautious explorative conservative surgery of solid tumors for lesions over 4 cm in diameter cannot, however, be accomplished without defining the tumor limits and exclusion of microinvasion of the tumor into the host capsule and adjacent kidney parenchyma. The adequacy of tumor resection would probably make more lesions amenable to partial nephrectomy by in situ techniques and ex vivo surgery on the work bench reserved for few selected complex central lesions. One uncertainty concerning nephron-sparing renal surgery is determination of the borders between healthy and tumorous tissues. Having an agent for localization of renal cell carcinoma and possibly cleaning tumor cells could make the argument for broader utilization of techniques of partial nephrectomy easier. In this study we made use of a new

[1] Chirurgische Universitätsklinik, Abteilung Urologie, Im Neuenheimer Feld 110, D-69120 Heidelberg, Germany
[2] Deutsches Krebsforschungszentrum, Im Neuenheimer Feld 280, D-69120 Heidelberg, Germany

class of photosensitizers for the laser-induced fluorescence diagnosis (LIFD) to investigate whether the surroundings of the eliminated renal tumor are free from tumor cells.

Previously the difficulty was to find photosensitizing compounds which are selectively accumulated in the tumor when injected systemically. Although several potentially useful photosensitizers on porphyrin and phtalocyanine bases are available, none is tumor specific. Clinical PDT to date has utilized either HpD, a mixture of at least nine porphyrin compounds [7], or dihematoporphyrin ether (DHE). No known photosensitizing drug is taken up or retained selectively only by malignant tissue. The purpose of this study was to evaluate the recently developed photosensitizing drug ‘PEOM’ (European patent pending, registered under PCT/EP91/00992) for its efficacy as photosensitizer for LIFD and PDT of renal cell carcinoma.

PEOM is a synthetic macromolecular bound derivative of porphyrin (molecular weight 15/20 kDa). This new system, consisting of a macromolecular carrier and photosensitizer drug, was developed as a result of experimental investigations in the search for photosensitizers which enable a labeling with indium-111 and also radioiodine. The carrier shows the following properties: (a) low clearance in kidney (high molecular weight compounds); (b) no or low trapping in the liver (below 15% of the dose applied); (c) long circulation half-life (6–8 days); (d) hydrophility, i.e., high capacity to bind water in the tumor interstitium; and (e) low catabolism rate in the tissues. The carrier was specially designed to be able to channel different low molecular compounds into the tumor [8]. We employed PEOM for treatment of human renal cell carcinoma xenotransplanted in nude mice. In view of the as yet limited experience with the use of PDT for therapy of this cancer, we made use of this experimental model to test PEOM as a tumor-localizing and actively photosensitizing agent for renal cell carcinoma tissue.

Materials and Methods

The model of subcapsular renal tumor xenotransplantation in mice was used. The tumor material of four patients nephrectomized at the Urology Department of the University of Heidelberg was employed. Fresh tumor specimens were freed from connective tissue and necrotic parts and cut up. Fragments approximately 1 mm in diameter were transplanted under the renal capsule of nude mice [9] by a special device [10] (Fig. 1). PEOM was injected intraperitoneally (0.5 μg/g body weight) into the mice 6–8 days after tumor transplantation. On the 18th day after transplantation, the tumors reached a diameter of 3–4 mm. Seven days after administration of the drug the tumor-bearing kidney was irradiated percutaneously with a total light dose of 2×60 J/cm^2 and a power density in the irradiated area of less than 150 mW/cm^2. A continuous-beam argon-pumped dye laser (656 nm) was used. For the distribution study of

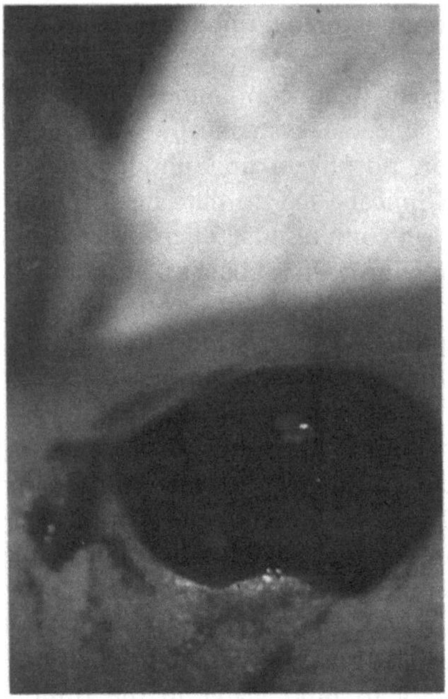

Fig. 1. Tumor tissue immediately after transplantation under the renal capsule in the left mouse kidney ×7; tumor size about 1 × 1 mm

PEOM, ^{131}I-labeled PEOM was injected simultaneously with the nonlabeled compound (1.85 MBq, 50 μCi).

Results

After the treatment with PEOM, the contents of the photosensitizer in tumor tissue lowered according to the level of tissue damage. Some 20%–30% of the administered dose was detected in the neoplastic tissue within 6–8 days post-injection. After excitation with laser light (488–514 nm), the vital tumor clusters and the surrounding tissues invaded with tumor cells showed intense red coloration by laser-induced fluorescence (Figs. 2–4). Subsequent to the light exposure (656 nm), a heavy tumor necrosis resulted, of up to 3–5 mm. No phototoxicity of surrounding normal tissue was observed. It took another 10 days for the edema and exudative reaction to subside (Fig. 5). As shown by the photographic documentation (Fig. 6), the neoplastic lesion disappeared and was replaced by a scar. The biopsy confirmed the therapeutic result. Generally, no toxicity of PEOM at a dose of up to 100 mg/kg body weight had been seen in previous pilot experiments.

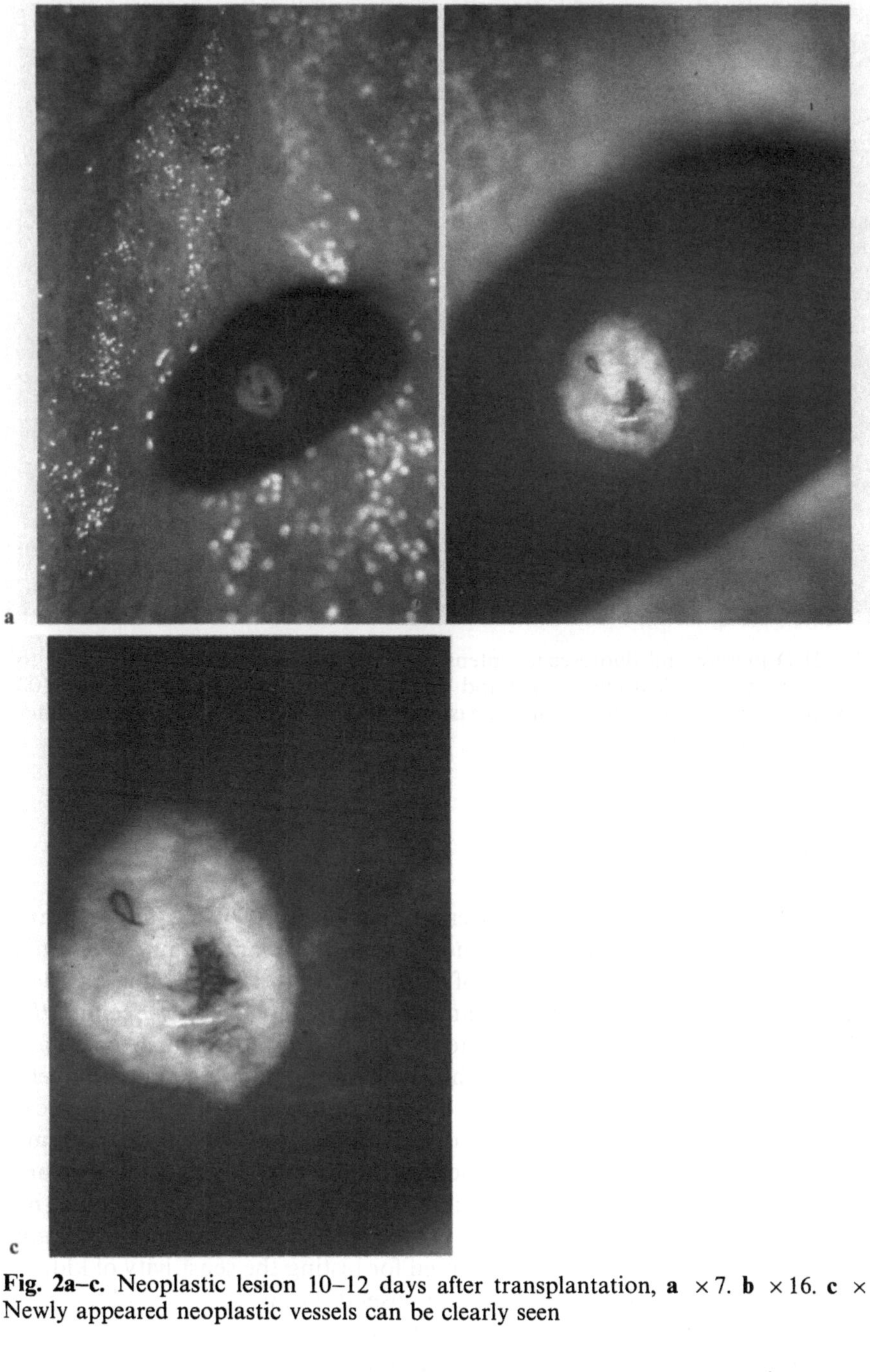

Fig. 2a–c. Neoplastic lesion 10–12 days after transplantation, **a** ×7. **b** ×16. **c** ×36. Newly appeared neoplastic vessels can be clearly seen

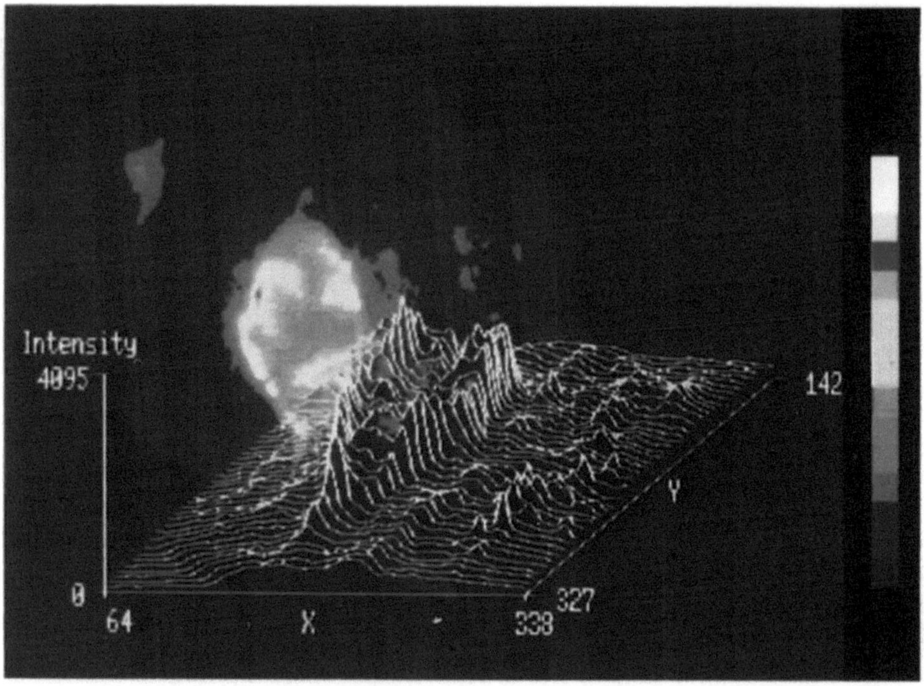

Fig. 3. LIFD picture and fluorescence intensity of the kidney with the tumor prior to PDT taken by the surgical microscope and single photon counting camera Argus 100 (Hamamatsu); excitation 400–514 nm; measured fluorescence with interference filter combination 690–720 nm

Discussion

We have shown in our treatment attempt that laser PDT has a significant antitumor effect on human adenocarcinoma xenotransplanted under the renal capsule of nude mice. The mechanism of its sensitivity to PDT demonstrated in this model can be explained by the damage of new blood vessels feeding the implanted tumor; the first was seen to be formed on the fourth day after transplantation. It is possible that the photosensitizer content in the tumor cells has some influence on the inhibition of tumor growth [10]. However, experiments performed with various tumors (sarcoma 180 and coloncarcinoma 173) have shown that the same treatment of tumors 10 days after transplantation, i.e., at a time when the neovascularization is established, resulted in no differences in the inhibition of tumor growth [10]. The subcapsular tumor xenotransplantation in mice kidney adapted for testing the sensitivity of kidney cancer to PDT proved to be especially useful because its histology and biological behavior resembles more the natural growth conditions of human renal cell carcinoma than the subcutaneous xenotransplants.

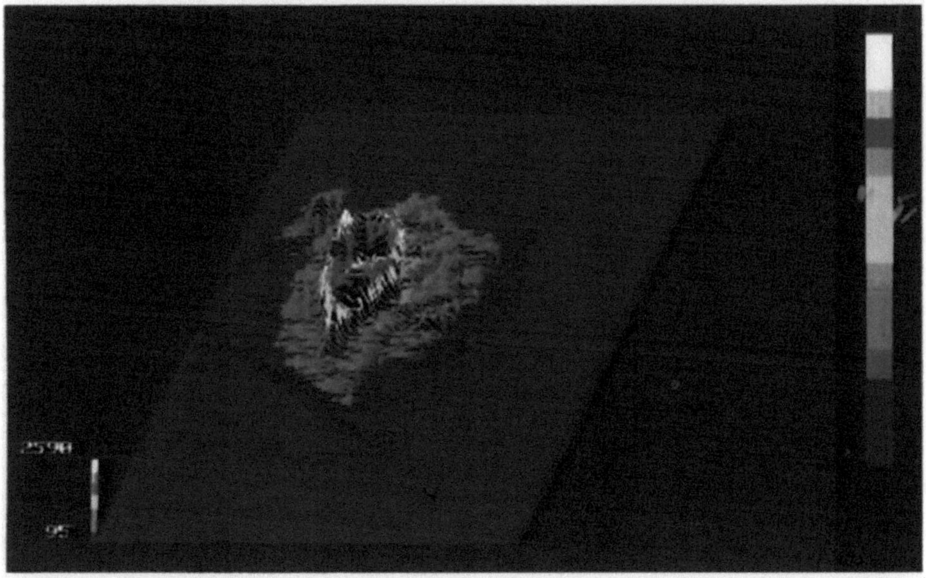

Fig. 4. Three-dimensional photosensitizer distribution in tumor and normal tissue; excitation 488–514 nm; emission 690–720 nm. *Dark blue* background

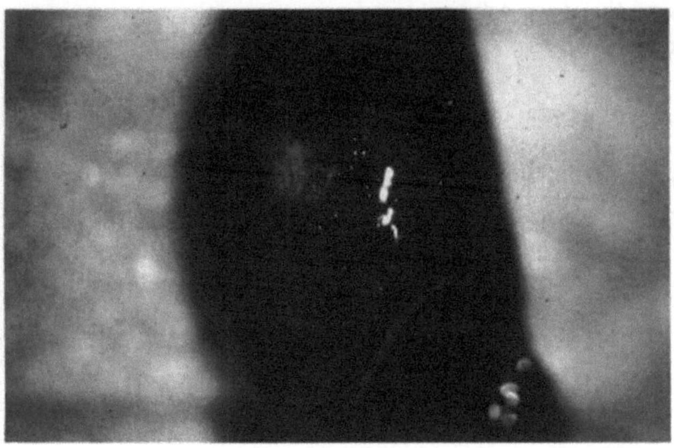

Fig. 5. Neoplastic lesion 12 days after PDT (× 16). The tumor has regressed; damage to the normal renal parenchyma is hardly recognizable. The intact renal capsule seems to be opaque

We believe that the newly developed macromolecular-derived porphyrin PEOM holds promise in the efficacy as photosensitizer. The high specific accumulation rate in the transplanted tumor was about 20%–30% of the dose administered as compared to only 0.2% to 3% for DHE. The accumulation ratio between tumor and normal tissue was generally better than 20:1. The

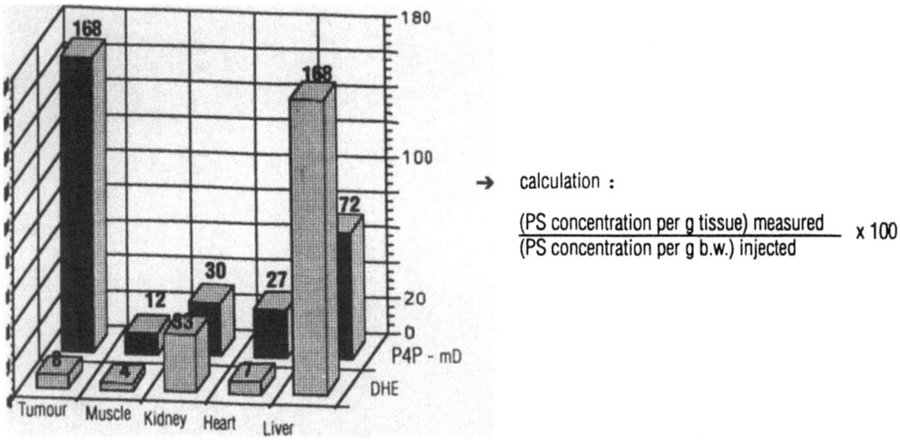

Fig. 6. Comparison of photosensitizer accumulation in five organs 3–7 days after drug administration. PEOM derivative P4P-mD (labeled with ^{131}I). DHE: labeled with ^{111}In

antitumor activity of PEOM was 20 times higher than that of DHE. The circulation time of PEOM was comparable to that of serum proteins. The clearance rate in the kidney was low (0.2–0.3 μg/g per hour). The trapping in the liver was approximately 15% lower than the liver accumulation of DHE, amounting to up to 60% of the dose administered.

We believe the future role of PDT in the management of tumors of the kidney is adjuvant within the concept of conservative kidney-preserving surgery. It seems that patient prognosis depends more on the adequacy of tumor resection [11, 12] and tumor stage [13] than on the fate of the contralateral kidney. Since the incomplete tumor excision carries a fatal danger for the patient [14], an extra safety margin of 1 cm can be achieved by erradication of tumor cells by PDT. Thus cure rates similar to those of radical nephrectomy can be expected.

References

1. Benson RC (1985) Treatment of diffuse transitional cell carcinoma in situ by whole bladder haematoporphyrin derivative photodynamic therapy. J Urol 134: 675–678
2. Jocham DS, Staehler G, Chaussy C, Hammer C, Lohrs U (1981) Laserbehandlung von Blasentumoren nach Photosensibilisierung mit Haematoporphyrin-Derivat. Urologe [A] 20: 340–345
3. Staehler G, Colombo M (1990) Laser ablation in urology. Lasers Med Sci 5: 203–207
4. Marberger M (1986) Conservative surgery for renal adenocarcinoma. In: de Kernion JB, Pavone-Macaluso M (eds) Tumors of the kidney. Williams and Wilkins, Baltimore
5. Novick AC, Streem S, Montie JE, Pontes JE, Siegel S, Montague DK, Goormastic U (1989) Conservative surgery for renal cell carcinoma. A single-center experience with 100 patients. J Urol 141: 835

6. Morgan WR, Zincke H (1990) Progression and survival after renal-conserving surgery for renal cell carcinoma: experience in 104 patients and extended follow up. J Urol 144: 852–858
7. Lipson RL, Blades EJ (1960) The photodynamic properties of a particular haematoporphyrin derivative. Arch Dermatol 82: 508–512
8. Sinn H, Schrenk HH, Friedrich EA, Schilling U, Maier-Borse W (1990) Design of a compound having an enhanced tumor uptake using serum albumin as a carrier, part I. Nucl Med Biol 17: 819–827
9. Bogden AE, Hasbell PM, Lepage DJ (1979) Growth of human xenografts implanted under the renal capsule of normal mice. Exp Cell Biol 17: 819–827
10. Graschev G, Shopova M, Anastassova G, Chakarova A, Getov C (1988) Sensitivity of individual tumors to photodynamic therapy. Lasers Med Sci 3: 233–238
11. Smith RB (1986) The treatment of bilateral renal cell carcinoma or renal cell carcinoma in the solitary kidney. In: de Kernion JB, Pavone-Macaluso M (eds) Tumors of the kidney. Williams and Wilkins, Baltimore
12. Jacobs SC, Berg S, Lawson RK (1980) Synchronous bilateral renal cell carcinoma; total surgical excision. Cancer 46: 234
13. Stöckle M, Störkel S, Mielke R, Steinbach F, Gallen E, Riedmiller H, Hohenfellner R (1990) Charakterisierung konservativ behandelter Nierenzellcarcinome. Aktuel Urol
14. Rosenthal CL, Kraft R, Zingg EJ (1984) Organ preserving surgery in renal cell carcinoma Tumor enucleation versus partial kidney resection. Eur Urol 10: 222–230

Subject Index

Springer-Verlag and the Environment

We at Springer-Verlag firmly believe that an international science publisher has a special obligation to the environment, and our corporate policies consistently reflect this conviction.

We also expect our business partners – paper mills, printers, packaging manufacturers, etc. – to commit themselves to using environmentally friendly materials and production processes.

The paper in this book is made from low- or no-chlorine pulp and is acid free, in conformance with international standards for paper permanency.

MIX
Papier aus verantwortungsvollen Quellen
Paper from responsible sources
FSC® C105338

If you have any concerns about our products,
you can contact us on
ProductSafety@springernature.com

In case Publisher is established outside the EU,
the EU authorized representative is:
Springer Nature Customer Service Center GmbH
Europaplatz 3, 69115 Heidelberg, Germany

Printed by Libri Plureos GmbH
in Hamburg, Germany